Practical Management of
ISCHAEMIC HEART DISEASE

PRACTICAL PROBLEMS IN MEDICINE

Practical Management of
ISCHAEMIC HEART DISEASE

Graham Jackson, FRCP
Consultant Cardiologist
King's College Hospital

Foreword by
Douglas A. Chamberlain,
MD FRCP
Consultant Cardiologist
Royal Sussex County Hospital
Brighton

MARTIN DUNITZ

© Graham Jackson, 1988

First published in the United Kingdom in 1988
by Martin Dunitz, 154 Camden High Street, London NW1 0NE

British Library Cataloguing in Publication Data

Jackson, Graham
  Practical management of ischaemic heart disease.
  — (Practical problems in medicine).
  1. Coronary heart disease
  I. Title   II. Series
  616.1′23   RC685.C6

  ISBN 0–948269–25–1

Phototypeset by Latimer Trend & Co. Ltd, Plymouth
Colour separations by Adroit Photolitho Ltd, Birmingham
Printed and bound in Singapore by Toppan Printing Company (S) Pte Ltd

For Maggie, Keira and Matthew

Acknowledgments

Most of the illustrations have been collected from patients under my care at King's College Hospital to whom I am grateful. Individuals are listed below in the publishers' acknowledgements; however I would like to extend my special thanks to my colleagues Fawaz Akhras, Stephen Campbell, Clifford Bucknall, John Chambers, and Mark Monaghan, to the nurses of the Coronary Unit, cardiac technicians and radiographers for collecting and helping me to prepare appropriate illustrations.

1988   G.J.

The publishers wish to acknowledge the following people for their help in the preparation of this book:

Stephen Campbell (Figure 5.9); Gower Medical Publishing Ltd (Figure 1.1, Figure 1.2, Figure 1.3, Figure 1.4, Figure 1.5); MCP Pharmaceuticals (Figure 5.3); Mark Monaghan (Figure 9.7, Figure 14.13, Figure 14.17); Vincent van Gogh Foundation/ National Museum Vincent van Gogh, Amsterdam (Figure 3.2); The Resuscitation Council UK (Figure 11.11); Reynolds Medical Ltd (Figure 19.1); Simonsen & Wheel Ltd (Figure 11.10).

Contents

Foreword

Ischaemic heart disease accounts for nearly half of all male deaths in Britain, and is an increasingly important cause in women. Fortunately, progress has been rapid over recent years in the development of treatments that alleviate symptoms and reduce mortality. Improvements in coronary surgery and percutaneous transluminal angioplasty, the expanding role of beta blockers, the reawaking of interest in antiplatelet agents, anticoagulants and thrombolytics, the evolving story of calcium channel blockers have all progressed at an almost breathless rate. In some countries—such as the United States—mortality has fallen substantially over a decade or more; new emphasis on prevention and better treatment may account for at least some of this change. What of Britain? Unfortunately we are beginning to lag seriously behind in the delivery of cardiological care to the community. The causes are manifold but include cost constraints, inadequate numbers of senior hospital posts in cardiology and cardiothoracic surgery and, related to this, uncertainty among the providers of primary health care with respect to what treatments can and should be offered to patients with symptomatic heart disease. Dr Jackson's book is therefore timely and will appeal particularly to general practitioners and to all those who need to know current views in this rapidly changing area. Dr Jackson's style reflects his penchant for teaching from his personal experience and is not a rehash of standard textbooks. The advice he offers is unashamedly personal but rarely idiosyncratic. It is didactic but supported by well chosen references. The book is unconventional, but it meets well an important need and is presented with flair. I wish it success.

DOUGLAS A. CHAMBERLAIN MD FRCP
Consultant Cardiologist
Royal Sussex County Hospital
Brighton

Preface

The purpose of this book is to provide a practical view of the management of the ischaemic patient. It is intended for family doctors but I hope may also be of help to junior doctors and students.

I have attempted to review current knowledge, which is not always scientifically secure, and based on this present the management in terms of 'what I do' or 'would do'. The need for a questioning attitude to clinical syndromes is essential and from this I have attempted to translate my approach into clearly reasoned guidelines of management. So where there is doubt I say so and then I commit myself based on what I believe is practical at present. I see no point in outlining arguments without reference to a clinical decision. Areas of doubt remain and so I recognize that opinions will change with time. However, this book is intended to be of help to those at the sharp end of patient care where we are faced with the need for immediate and longterm decision making designed for each *individual* patient.

References are included to support observations and as a guide for further study. I have attempted to be fair to past authors but if their key work is not referenced I can only apologize. Some might argue that to reference only one or two review articles is all that is needed but to depend entirely on reviews means depending entirely on the opinions of other authors. Given that this book is essentially my opinion it had to stem from the original works to be of any use to the reader.

I am greateful for the help and advice of my colleagues David Jewitt and Douglas Chamberlain. I also acknowledge the support of my junior staff and the kindness and patience of the publishers.

Finally my family deserve a mention for coping with my constant retreats to the study; their understanding and caring I hope has all been worthwhile.

1
Pathology

BACKGROUND

Angina, myocardial infarction, arrhythmias, and heart failure are the practical clinical consequences of myocardial ischaemia, and the most common pathological mechanism is obstructive coronary artery disease (CAD). In the presence of coronary atheroma, myocardial blood supply may fail to meet metabolic demands with the result that a shift occurs from aerobic to anaerobic metabolism. Other forms of supply/demand imbalance can independently result in myocardial ischaemia, and include hypertension and aortic valve disease. These are discussed as part of the differential diagnosis (see page 43). When considering the pathological basis for myocardial ischaemia and infarction, we are concerned principally with atheratomous plaques.

ATHEROMATOUS PLAQUES

There are two major forms of atheromatous plaque:

1 The fibrous plaque which is a white raised lesion, often concentric, which predominantly contains smooth muscle cells and no or minimal amounts of extracellular lipid (see Figure 1.1).
2 A lipid-rich plaque which is often eccentric. Here a fibrous cap formed from smooth muscle cells covers a softer 'porridge-like' centre containing cell debris and free lipid, emphasizing the proliferative and degenerative nature of the lesion (see Figure 1.2).

Both these lesions may exist in the same patient but it is the lipid-rich lesions which are more prone to haemorrhage, ulceration, and mural thrombosis, and thus have the potential for coronary occlusion.

AETIOLOGY

The exact mechanism for the development of coronary atheroma is not known. The response-to-injury[1,2] hypothesis states that in the presence of repeated injury, connective tissue elements will proliferate, bind lipoproteins, and the plaque will develop. Clinically recognizable sources of injury include:

- Cigarette smoking (toxic cell wall damage from carbon monoxide and platelet aggregation and lipid deposition in the arterial wall)
- Hypertension (haemodynamic injury, increased arterial well tension and permeability of the endothelium to lipids)
- Diabetes (hyperlipidaemia, increased lipid binding in the arterial wall)
- Obesity (diabetes, hypertension, increased cardiac work)
- Possible infective/immunological insult.[3]

Prostaglandins and platelets are also implicated.[4] The endothelium and intima produce prostacyclin from arachidonic acid which inhibits platelet aggregation; whereas thromboxane which is produced by aggregating platelets is a powerful vasoconstrictor which may cause platelets to aggregate further. Platelet damage can be superimposed on endothelial damage, thereby expanding the lesion.[5,6] Platelet-derived growth factor (PDGF) may then cause multiplication of cells within and adjacent to the original endothelial damage, expanding the lesion further.[7]

It has also been proposed that the plaque stems from a single smooth muscle cell (the monoclonal theory).[8] In support of this, it is known that early plaques have isoenzymatic markers of an identical chromosomal make-up. Could this cell then be altered, perhaps by injury, from a benign to a neoplastic lesion?

Our current knowledge can be summarized as an interaction between the endothelial cell and a series of varying traumas shown diagrammatically (Figure 1.3).

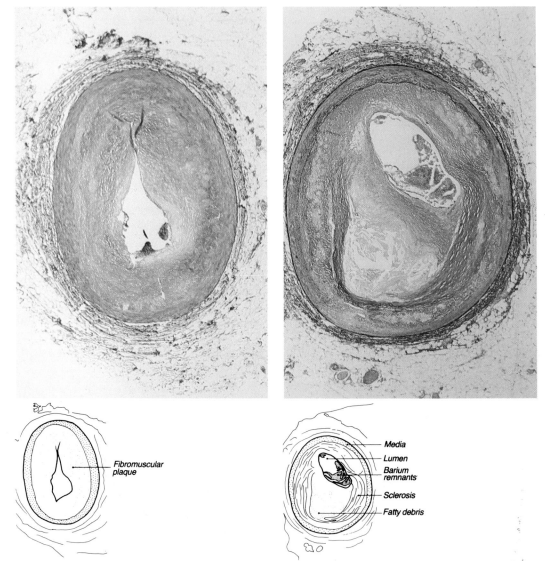

Figure 1.1 Section of coronary artery showing concentric narrowing due to atherosclerosis; the lesion is mainly composed of fibromuscular tissues rather than atheroma or dense collagen. Elastic-van Gieson stain.

Figure 1.2 Histological section of coronary artery showing classic atherosclerotic lesion. Fatty debris is the major plaque constituent. Elastic-van Gieson stain.

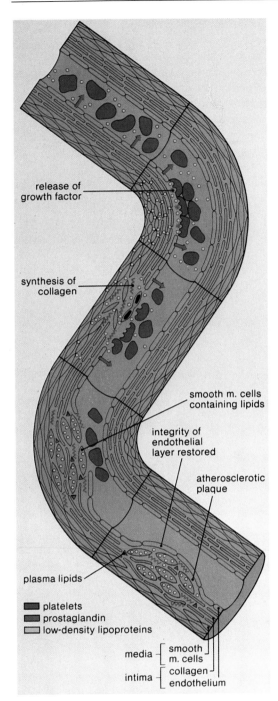

release of growth factor

synthesis of collagen

smooth m. cells containing lipids

integrity of endothelial layer restored

atherosclerotic plaque

plasma lipids

■ platelets
■ prostaglandin
□ low-density lipoproteins

media ⎡ smooth ⎤
⎣ m. cells ⎦

intima ⎡ collagen ⎤
⎣ endothelium ⎦

Figure 1.3 Segments of artery showing different stages of atherogenesis according to concept of Ross and Glomset.

CLINICAL SYNDROMES

Myocardial infarction

A myocardial infarction is death of myocardial tissue secondary to a loss of blood supply. Two pathological types are recognized: (1) regional infarction; (2) non-regional infarction.

REGIONAL INFARCTION The area of necrosis is directly related to an artery subtending the region of supply (Figure 1.4). It may be of variable size, depending on the artery involved and of full thickness (transmural) or subendocardial (non-transmural, also known as non-Q-wave). The presence of an alternative blood supply (collaterals) to the area involved will also affect the extent of damage.

Pathological studies in regional infarction have consistently identified occlusive thrombi in the anatomically predicted artery. A tear of 1–1.5 mm in the intimal fibrous cap of an underlying plaque is also usually found (Figure 1.5), and the thrombus may dissect into the intima both proximally and distally.

NON-REGIONAL INFARCTION This is also known as diffuse infarction. Necrosis occurs in the inner zone of the left ventricle. The ischaemia is global usually after a reduction in myocardial perfusion secondary to generalized proximal and distal CAD. It may therefore be seen more frequently in diabetics who are vulnerable to generalized atheroma, and present as an ischaemic fibrotic cardiomyopathy leading to arrhythmias and heart failure. Although thrombi may be found in small vessels, they are not implicated in initiating a non-regional infarction.

Because of the varying nature of atheroma, regional and non-regional infarction may coexist in the same patient and non-regional necrosis may occur secondary to regional necrosis if the infarct is extensive and complicated by a major drop in blood pressure, as in cardiogenic shock.

3

MUSCLE DAMAGE

Most infarcts affect the left ventricle; right ventricular infarction, however, is seen frequently enough to suggest that the pathological involvement of the right ventricle, particularly with inferior infarcts, may be more frequent than is realized (see page 109).

In experimental coronary occlusion studies, cell death occurs within 60 minutes which gives little time for salvage procedures. The infarct area initially looks pale and glossy becoming yellowish at 24 hours. At the cellular level, coagulation necrosis occurs (cytoplasmic eosinophilia and nuclear pyknosis) with mitochondrial swelling and sarcolemma damage as the earliest signs. At 24 hours, light microscopic changes include clumping of the cytoplasm of myocardial fibres, alteration in cross striations, nuclear blurring, and leucocyte (mainly neutrophils) proliferation.

An infarct at seven days is yellow with a peripheral hyperaemic zone. The white cells decrease in the second week and from three to

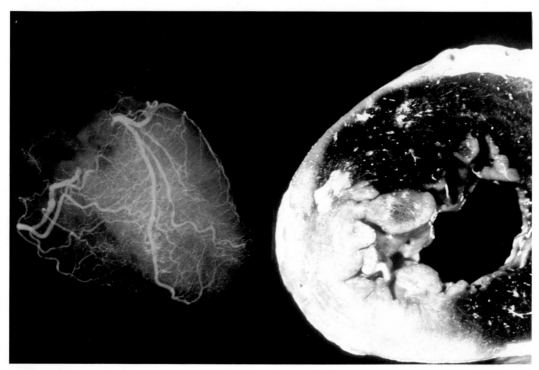

Figure 1.4 (left) Port-mortem coronary angiogram showing major obstruction in left marginal branch; (right) transmural infarct confined to area supplied by obstructed artery. Nitro blue tetrazolium technique (viable muscle stains dark blue).

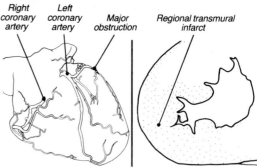

Right coronary artery   Left coronary artery   Major obstruction   Regional transmural infarct

five days phagocytosis occurs. At two weeks, muscle renewal progresses to an advanced stage with scar formation progressing over four to six weeks, to complete healing around six weeks with a sclerotic, almost acellular scar. At this point the infarct is thin and pale grey in colour. Although this is the usual time-scale, variations exist and depend on the size of the infarction, presence of complications, and extent of collateral blood supply.

THROMBOSIS

While clinical and pathological studies have identified thrombus in the coronary artery supplying an area of acute infarction, controversy has surrounded the sequence of events—namely, did the thrombus cause the infarct or was it secondary? It is now believed that in the majority of cases the prime cause of acute regional infarction is occlusion of the artery secondary to acute coronary arterial thrombosis.[9,10]

This argument has been strengthened by placebo-controlled studies of streptokinase in which the lytic agent reduced infarct size, decreased mortality, and increased arterial patency when given at the time of coronary occlusion (within 4 to 6 hours of infarction).[11,12]

Thrombosis usually follows plaque rupture at areas of greater than 50 per cent luminal narrowing (see Figure 1.5).[13] This is a complication of the lipid-rich plaques. A small tear may give rise to a massive thrombus in those with an increased thrombotic tendency but usually there is a rupture greater than 1 cm so that flowing blood comes into contact with lipid and a propagating thrombus follows. The cause of plaque rupture is unknown.

ANGINA

Most patients with stable angina have fixed obstructive coronary atheroma. A reduction of 70 per cent in cross-sectional area of the lumen reduces exertional flow and a 95 per cent reduction reduces flow at rest. Lesions are often found in the larger parts of the proximal epicardial coronary arteries, frequently at sites of bifurcation. Plaques may be lipid-rich, fibrous, or both.

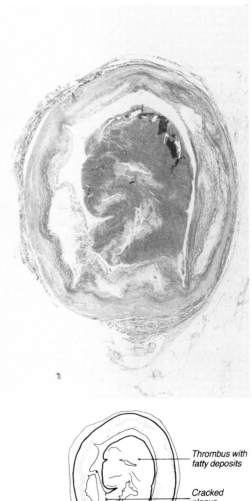

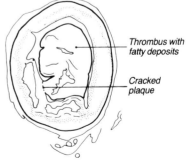

Thrombus with fatty deposits

Cracked plaque

Figure 1.5 Histological section of coronary artery with cracked plaque and adherent thrombus containing fatty debris from the plaque. Elastic-van Gieson stain.

5

The presence of arterial spasm superimposed on these lesions may render the angina unstable. For this to occur, vasoactive materials must be released from platelets leading to arterial vasoconstriction, and would need a disruption of endothelial integrity by atheroma, intact smooth muscle cells to facilitate constriction, and areas of disease without a satisfactory collateral supply.

A feature of many patients with angina is the absence of significant muscular damage.

SUDDEN DEATH

This may occur at the time of acute infarction but also without any evidence of infarction. In 70 per cent of patients the cause is related to CAD. The presence of plaque fissures and large or small intraluminal thrombi suggest a sudden ischaemic event quite separate from the stable angina picture.[13] Perhaps the ischaemic event leads to a change from aerobic to anaerobic metabolism at such a speed that ventricular fibrillation precedes infarction, ie, they would have infarcted if time had allowed and there had been no intervention.

CORONARY ARTERY BYPASS GRAFTS

The atheroma that develops in the bypasses is the same as that in the native vessels, and death similarly follows plaque rupture, ulceration and thrombosis. The skill of the surgeon in avoiding turbulence at the anastomosis (response-to-injury) is important, as is the avoidance of risk factors in the postoperative period.[14]

ANGIOPLASTY

Balloon dilatation of narrow coronary arteries has become a major new therapeutic option for the ischaemic patient. The plaque may be forced out into the media, or the media opposite may be stretched. Thrombosis is the greatest problem when lipid-rich particles come into contact with blood rather than being forced outwards, and this occurs more frequently with eccentric lipid-rich plaques which may dissect. Correct positioning of the balloon across the lesion, preventing distal spread of the flattened plaque and its contents (ie, ensuring they are forced into the wall), appears fundamental to the safety of the procedure.

PRACTICAL POINTS

- Atheromatous plaques remain the greatest cause of ischaemic cardiac events.

- Myocardial infarction invariably follows an acute thrombosis caused by plaque rupture.

- Muscle damage usually relates directly to the vessel occluded and appears irreversible in 3–4 hours.

- Angina is caused in most patients by fixed obstructive coronary arterial disease.

- Unstable angina appears to fall between stable angina and myocardial infarction with a variable amount of plaque fissuring and vasoconstriction.

2
Epidemiology (risk factors)

BACKGROUND

Epidemiology is the study of the distribution and determinants of disease by examining samples of populations rather than individual clinical problems. Certain characteristics in healthy individuals have been strongly associated with the subsequent development of coronary artery disease (CAD).

Although these 'risk factors' are closely associated with the disease, they are not necessarily directly related to the development of atherosclerosis, ie, they are not definitely causative. They are indicators of risk, whether direct or indirect. Specific management of risk factors is discussed later (see page 23).

SCALE OF THE PROBLEM

Cardiovascular disease is responsible for 50 per cent of the deaths of men aged forty-five to fifty-four years and 40 per cent of those between thirty-five and forty-four years (see Figure 2.1). Each year in England and Wales 160 000 men and women die from coronary heart disease and 25 per cent are below sixty-five years of age. At the 1984 rates 9 per cent of all men will die from coronary heart disease by sixty-five and 19 per cent by seventy-five years. Abolishing this would allow 800 more men in 10 000 to reach retirement age even allowing for other diseases.[1]

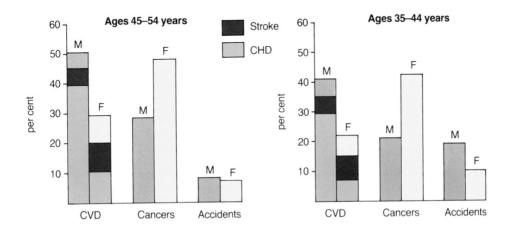

Figure 2.1 Coronary heart disease (CHD) mortality represents the major proportion of cardiovascular (CVD) deaths. Although it increases with age it still represents the major cause of death in men (M) between thirty-five and forty-four years of age.

The disease in the community can also be expressed as working days lost. Premature male cardiac deaths account for 250 000 lost working days each year and some 200 million working days are lost because of illness from ischaemic heart disease (IHD). This represents approximately 8 per cent of all days lost and is a greater percentage than that from all industrial disputes combined.[2]

The average family doctor in the UK (list 2500) will lose seven patients a year from his list as a result of IHD. Since 20 per cent of men sustain an infarct before retiring, 100 post-infarct patients will be on the list. In the age range forty-five to sixty-four years there will

be thirteen in 1000 consultations for cardiac infarction, twelve in 1000 for angina, thirteen in 1000 for other IHD, seven in 1000 for cerebrovascular disease, and seven in 1000 for peripheral vascular disease. By combining the figures for peripheral and cerebral vascular disease with those for CAD on a national scale we can identify 200 000 atheromatous deaths out of a total of 580 000 annual deaths,[3] and therefore the need and scope for prevention should be treated with some urgency.

GEOGRAPHICAL INCIDENCE

Mortality from coronary heart disease varies from country to country[4] (see Figure 2.2) but there are also regional variations within countries.[5]

Within the UK the regional variation is striking, with a rising gradient of risk from the south east to the north west and Scotland. This remains significant after allowing for social class factors (see Figure 2.3). Scotland now has one of the highest mortalities from coronary heart disease in the world. In the USA the highest incidence is along the east coast, in the industrial Mid-West, and in the north east. In Europe trends show a similar rising pattern from the less industrialized areas (Italy, Greece) to the more industrial countries.

Although the differences could be attributed to varying diagnostic criteria, the range is too great for this to be the sole reason, and in the UK, where this is not applicable, there is a genuine variation within the regions.

MORTALITY TRENDS

While there has been no convincing reduction in coronary heart disease mortality in the UK, there are some signs of this happening in those under forty-five years[6] and deaths in the professional classes have fallen.[7] In contrast, there has been a dramatic fall in death from coronary heart disease in the USA in all groups, male and female. Between 1968 and

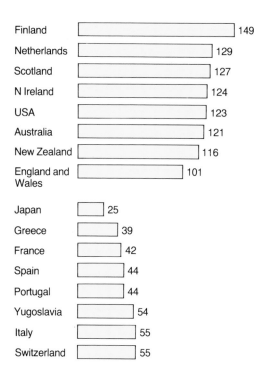

Figure 2.2 Mortality index per 100 000 (men aged 45–54 years) from different countries (1971). The rate in Scotland has now increased to similar levels to those in Finland.

8

1977 the USA death rate fell 20 per cent (see Figure 2.4) verging on the unchanged rate for England and Wales.

It is known that mortality rates for men are greater than for women (see Figure 2.5) and are most marked in middle age. The rates merge around sixty-five years (approximately fifteen years after the menopause). Women generally show the same geographical pattern but unlike men death from heart disease in women has declined in England and Wales.[8]

Looking at the high-risk group of men between forty-five and sixty-four years, an interesting pattern emerges. Data from Canada[9] show similar patterns to the USA and a decreased mortality has been recorded for Australia and New Zealand. In Finland[10] mortality has decreased most rapidly in north Karelia whereas in Sweden[11], with similar lifestyle changes, there has been no decline and even evidence of a rise.

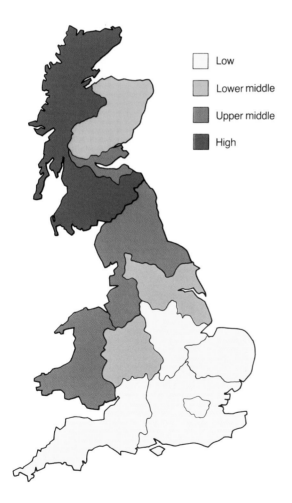

Low

Lower middle

Upper middle

High

Figure 2.3 Regional differences in coronary heart disease in men aged forty-five to fifty-four years.

Why the change?

That there has has been a change in some parts of the world is most encouraging. If clear-cut reasons for declining mortality could be identified, the opportunities for widespread prevention might be enormous. There is no doubt that there has been a fall in mortality rates in the USA but no single factor has been identified. It could simply be a natural lengthening of biological age, which would have a major impact on a chronic disease state; it may reflect increased nutrition and better control of environmental and infectious disease problems. If there has been a decrease in the extent of CAD the impact should have been greater in the younger age group but in the USA the benefit crosses all ages, both sexes, and black and white races.[12]

It is possible to attribute the improvements to better treatment, reduced smoking habits, improved identification of hypertension and better therapy, dietary changes, and increased physical activity. Women have, however, continued to smoke and still received benefit, and the greatest benefit has occurred in black women. Whilst better blood pressure control could be effective, it is difficult to attribute this to changing smoking patterns (blacks

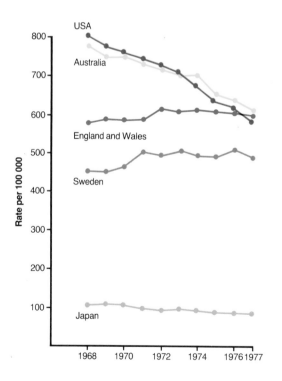

Figure 2.4 Changes in heart disease mortality. There is a decrease in the USA and Australia in contrast with the statistics in England and Wales.

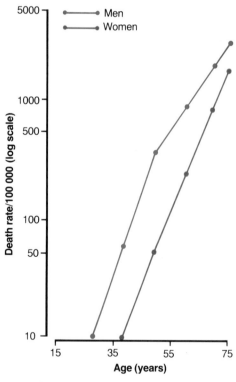

Figure 2.5 Mortality rates for men and women.

smoke less than whites) and increased exercise (black women exercise less). Diet has changed little in the UK while in Australia and the USA the ratio of polyunsaturated fat to saturated fat has altered. This overall change has occurred in Sweden, however, which has an increase in heart disease, and furthermore no diet change or increase in saturated fat in Japan and Switzerland[13] is associated with a decrease in heart disease.

While a decrease in smoking as an independent variable shows a correlation with a change in heart disease mortality, it may also be a component of social class changes. A decreased incidence of heart disease in classes I and II (professional) compared with IV and V (working) may reflect falling cigarette consumption in classes I and II and perhaps varying dietary factors. It remains of interest that the only group in the UK identified as showing a fall in mortality are doctors, who are from the professional classes and who now smoke less.[14]

Summarizing these observations, it seems that a build up of a variety of risks is responsible for the development of coronary heart disease, and studies indicate that the population would benefit from a general reduction in risk factors rather than a specific isolated change. It is important to note, however, that the downward trend in the USA preceded many of the current lifestyle changes.

Family history

There is no doubt that all doctors are aware of families of patients with coronary heart disease. Certainly with the inherited hyperlipidaemias there is clear evidence of a genetic factor, but this only affects about one in 250 of the general population and therefore cannot be implicated in most cases.[15]

Studies in South Africa and the USA have shown wide variations in heart disease between racial groups within a single country. In addition there is wide variation between various countries with Japan experiencing a remarkably low mortality rate from coronary heart disease—of the order of 10 per cent of the UK rate. There may therefore appear to be a genetic basis for disease which responds to environmental factors, or it could simply be a variation in environment that affects coronary risk.

Japanese emigrants[16] who have lived long enough in their new environment (USA) resemble native Americans in coronary disease incidence. Similar observations have been recorded for other migratory groups. We do not experience migration from wealthy to poor areas so the reverse data are not available, though during a time of poverty and malnutrition in the 1940–45 war and shortly afterwards, atheromatous diseases are believed to have fallen even allowing for problems with data recording. The Japanese who maintain their traditional lifestyle in a new environment do not show an increase in coronary heart disease. However, this is most likely the first-generation migrant and developments should be looked for in the younger generation who were raised from youth or childhood in the higher risk Western setting.

Before the recent fall in the incidence of coronary heart disease in the USA, a significant rise had been noted from the early post-war years within a given population group. The suggestion of a predominance of environmental and cultural factors in the aetiology of coronary heart disease refutes genetic markers as the major prevention prospect for the future.

RISK FACTORS

Three major risk factors have been identified:

- Smoking
- Hypertension
- Raised serum cholesterol.

Addition of factors

At present it is safe to say that there is no

single cause of coronary atheroma. We know that various factors—risk factors—are associated with coronary heart disease and are possibly causative. In addition these factors are synergistic (see Figure 2.6).

In the American Pooling Project[17] men aged between thirty and fifty-nine years who smoked cigarettes doubled the risk of having an infarct. When hypertension (diastolic blood pressure > 90 mmHg) or raised cholesterol (> 6.5 mmol/l; 250 mg/100 ml) levels coexisted the risk rose four times but with all three it rose eight-fold.

Many other factors (see Table 2.1) play a part, some of which are avoidable and some which are not (eg, age, sex and family history). Given an unavoidable risk it becomes more imperative for the patient and physician to modify the avoidable risks. It is unusual to possess one risk factor to a high degree (eg, inherited hyperlipidaemia) and more common to have a mild or moderate degree of more than one risk factor. It is worth noting the cumulative risk of the three major factors (see Figure 2.7).

Smoking

All forms of smoking are associated with increased incidence of IHD but cigarettes are more dangerous than cigars or a pipe.[18] Cigarette smoking is responsible for 25 per cent of all coronary deaths in men and women aged sixty-five years or less and 80 per cent of men below forty-five years. This means that 10 000 men and women of less than sixty-five years die annually from coronary heart disease as a result of cigarette smoking. The risk of a fatal coronary event is three times greater

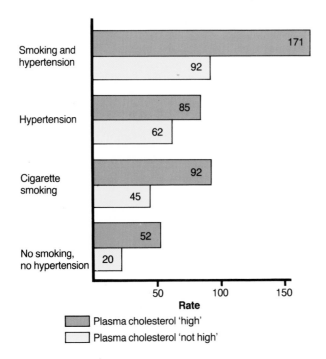

Figure 2.6 Additive effects of three major risk factors related to cholesterol levels.

than that for a non-smoker, but in the group of men less than forty-five years who smoke over twenty cigarettes a day the risk is fifteen times higher than for the non-smoker (see Figure 2.8). The more cigarettes smoked the greater this risk is for all age groups, although the incidence always rises with age.[19]

It is important to note that individuals who stop smoking have a substantial and rapid reduction of risk from heart attack and sudden death[14] (see Figure 2.9; see also Chapter 3), while those who continue to smoke after a heart attack have double the risk of a fatal or non-fatal relapse.

Although most studies show a close link between smoking and coronary heart disease, the Japanese form an exception. Japanese men smoke an average of fifteen to twenty cigarettes a day compared with ten to fifteen in the UK and have a significant incidence of hypertension, yet their coronary mortality is one-tenth that of the UK.

Table 2.1   Risk factors

Major	Minor
Increasing age	Obesity
Male sex	Stress
Cigarette smoking	Soft water
Hypertension	Hyperuricaemia
Hypercholesterolaemia	
Diabetes	

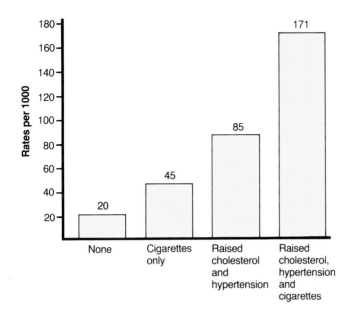

Figure 2.7   Additive effect of risk factors on the incidence of a first major coronary event.

The Japanese, however, have very low cholesterol levels and eat a lot of fatty fish which might protect them, ie, smoking needs the bed of dietary indiscretion to exert its most harmful effects. In all other groups it remains a powerful independent risk factor for coronary heart disease.

There is a clear relationship between smoking and the degree of coronary disease[20] as well as a history of infarction.[21] But infarction may be independent of the severity of stenoses (ie, occur in mild disease) raising the dual threat of smoking causing both atherosclerosis and acutely precipitating infarction by an additional mechanism (eg, thrombosis).

MECHANISM The exact mechanism of cigarette toxicity is unknown.[22] We do know that cigarettes contain two potentially toxic agents, nicotine and carbon monoxide.[23] The amount of nicotine inhaled varies between the so-called non-inhaler and the deep inhaler. The latter may absorb up to 100 mg a day. Nicotine stimulates catecholamine production with a resultant rise in heart rate, blood pressure and cardiac contraction, ie, increased oxygen demand. In addition there is an increased tendency to platelet aggregation, increased fibrinogen, and free fatty acids with a decrease in insulin secretion and a tendency to hyperglycaemia.

At the same time as demand is rising, supply is falling because of the inhalation of carbon monoxide. Cigarette smoke contains up to 6 per cent carbon monoxide with an air content of eight times the allowable industrial level. Because of the haemoglobin's greater affinity for carbon monoxide versus oxygen (200 times) the oxygen content is decreased. In the presence of atheroma the normal response of increasing coronary blood flow to compensate is limited.[23]

Cigarette smoking increases the myocardial workload by catecholamine stimulation at the same time as it reduces oxygen supply by carbon monoxide inhalation. Low tar cigarettes confer no benefit and the risk is equally important for men and women.[24]

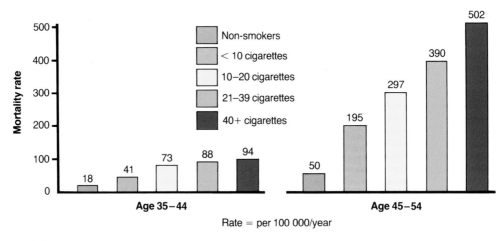

Figure 2.8 Mortality for coronary heart disease in men who smoke.

LIPIDS

Cholesterol

One of the most useful population studies is that of Japanese men living in Japan, Hawaii, and Los Angeles.[16] In Japan the calorie intake as fat is 13 per cent and the mean cholesterol level is 3.9 mmol/l (150 mg/100 ml). In Los Angeles 40 per cent of the calories are as fat and the mean cholesterol is 6.5 mmol/l (250 mg/100 ml). Ischaemic heart disease is ten times more frequent in Los Angeles than in Japan. In Hawaii the levels for diet, cholesterol, and IHD were intermediate. These changes occurred independently of other risk factors which were evenly distributed.

The Seven Countries Study[25], which followed 12 000 men aged between forty and fifty years for ten years, reported a strong relationship between a serum cholesterol level of over 5.7 mmol/l (222 mg/100 ml) and the development of IHD.

Those with a cholesterol greater than 7.75 mmol/l (300 mg/100 ml) had a three-fold greater risk of an infarct compared with those with a level of 5.8 mmol/l (225 mg/100 ml) or less.

One of the problems of establishing a normal range for cholesterol levels is that we have no clear idea of what is normal. Within the range 3.6–7.75 mmol/l (140–300 mg/100 ml) there is a graded risk and it is obviously better to be at the lower end of the range. In practical terms it is easy to be complacent about a normal report but closer scrutiny is needed because so-called 'normal' is not necessarily safe or right. It is better to be more normal than just normal.

The Pooling Project Research Group[17] derived from eight longterm studies on 12 381 men in the USA showed a greater increase in IHD with higher levels of total serum cholesterol (see Figure 2.10). The optimal level for risk appeared to be around 5.4 mmol/l (210 mg/100 ml). The possibility of increased non-cardiac deaths, eg, from cancer in the low-cholesterol group, has been a cause for concern, but in this study there was no excess

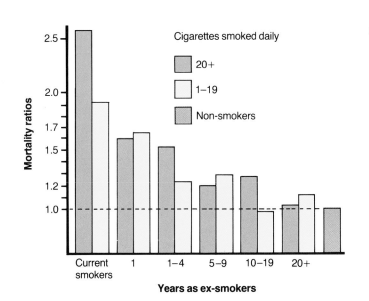

Figure 2.9 Effect of stopping smoking.

15

of non-cardiac deaths in the low-cholesterol groups, and in the Mediterranean countries where fat provides 25–30 per cent of dietary energy and with a mean cholesterol of 4.5 mmol/l (174 mg/100 ml) total morbidity and mortality from cancer was lower than in the UK or USA.

The most powerful evidence of a link between cholesterol and IHD stems from studies of familial hypercholesterolaemia which show an independent risk for IHD up to ten-fold.[15]

Lipoproteins

The varying lipid-bearing particles in plasma (lipoproteins) also seem to be linked to the development of IHD.[26]

The lipoprotein fractions are:

- Chylomicrons
- Very low density lipoproteins (VLDL)
- Low density lipoproteins (LDL)
- High density lipoproteins (HDL).

The lipids are triglycerides which act as energy carriers and storage substrates (excess of food stored in fatty tissue); cholesterol which is a component of cell walls required for new membranes during cell division and maintenance of membrane function; and phospholipids which are essential for the development of subcellular structures. The lipids are not water soluble but are changed to a soluble transport form by being bound to specific protein bodies (apoproteins). The resulting large molecular complex is the lipoprotein.

1 **VERY LOW DENSITY LIPOPROTEINS** These are mainly synthesised in the liver, transport triglycerides to adipose tissues, and when depleted become smaller and smaller. They become richer in cholesterol and phospholipids and finally become the small cholesterol-rich LDL.

2 **LOW DENSITY LIPOPROTEINS** These carry cholesterol from adipose tissue to cells. About 45 per cent of circulatory cholesterol is in this form and a further 30 per cent is in an intermediate form (IDL).

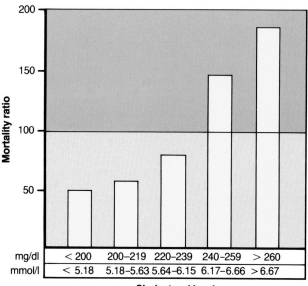

Figure 2.10 Coronary heart disease and cholesterol. Increased risk with rising cholesterol levels.

3 **HIGH DENSITY LIPOPROTEINS** These are formed in the liver and contain 30 per cent phospholipids and 20 per cent cholesterol. They take up cholesterol freed from cells and return it to the HDL pool.

4 **CHYLOMICRONS** These transport fats absorbed from the intestine and are normally detected in the digestive phase. They leave remnants which transport cholesterol from adipose tissue to the liver for storage and redistribution.

The risk of heart disease appears to rise with increasing LDL and VLDL[27] (see Table 2.2) but the risk of IHD in both sexes is lower with high levels of HDL and the ratio of HDL:total cholesterol and especially HDL:LDL provides a sensitive index of risk (see Table 2.3).

While raised LDL and reduced HDL are independently associated with coronary heart disease, VLDL emerges as a risk factor in some studies but not an independent one. In adults LDL levels below 3.4 mmol/l (130 mg/100 ml), HDL levels above 1.3 mmol/l (50 mg/100 ml) and total cholesterol:HDL ratios below five are targets for reduced risk.[28,29]

High density lipoprotein cholesterol levels are positively related to exercise and moderate alcohol intake, and inversely related to cigarette smoking, obesity and the contraceptive pill. Similarly various drugs affect the lipid profiles (see Table 2.4). Familial excess of HDL (hyperalphalipoproteinaemia) or deficiency of LDL (hypobetalipoproteinaemia) is associated with decreased coronary heart disease risk and longevity.[15]

Table 2.2 Lipoproteins and risk

	Protein per cent	Cholesterol per cent	Triglycerides per cent	Phospholipids per cent	Risk
Chylomicrons	2	7	85	6	Low
VLDL	7	20	55	18	High
LDL	21	47	9	23	Very high
HDL	47	18	7	28	Protection

Table 2.3 'Protective' effect of increasing HDL cholesterol (Framingham)[3]

HDL–cholesterol level mg/100ml	Rate of coronary events per 1000	
	Men	Women
< 34	107	155
35–54	79	51
> 55	43	27

Cholesterol conversion: mmol/litre × 38.7 = mg/100 ml.

The lipid abnormalities have been classified by Fredrickson into five groups (see Table 2.5). The most common groups associated with IHD are types II with predominantly hypercholesterolaemia, type IV with hypertriglyceridaemia and IIb with a mixture. Type IIa and b may be inherited whereas type IV is frequently linked to obesity, diabetes, renal failure and alcoholism.

Future prospects for further risk definition will involve the protein constituents of the lipoproteins. A decreased plasma apo-1 (major part of HDL) or an increased apo-B (part of LDL) may serve as important and better risk factors than LDL and HDL cholesterol. Similarly HDL_2, the cholesterol-rich subfraction of HDL, may also prove a better risk predictor.[15,17]

For the present raised total cholesterol is a definite independent risk factor for CAD. The total cholesterol: HDL ratio is a useful additive index.

Hypertension

Raised blood pressure increases the risk of coronary heart disease in both men and women.[17,30] Severe hypertension may present with cerebrovascular accidents and heart failure whereas mild to moderate hypertension relates to coronary heart disease.[31] The greatest risk is above 100 mmHg diastolic and the average general practice will contain fifty middle-aged men with such a reading. Hypertension increases with age and its importance as a risk factor persists. As mild hypertension is undiagnosed in 40 per cent of the population this contributes significantly to CAD. A blood pressure of over 160/95 mmHg leads to a three-fold chance of CAD, seven-fold risk of stroke, four to seven-fold chance of heart failure, and a three-fold chance of peripheral arterial disease. This risk is in addition to other major risk factors (see Figure 2.6).

Diabetes

In western industrialized societies diabetics are more likely to develop coronary heart disease,[32] the incidence being the same for both sexes. Even in Japan with its low incidence of coronary heart disease the risk is higher in diabetics. Furthermore the mortality after infarction is 50 per cent in one year (in non-diabetics it is less than 10 per cent).

Table 2.4 Effects of drugs (other than specific lipid-lowering agents) on lipid levels

Drug	Cholesterol	HDL	Triglycerides
Beta-blockers	↑	↓	↑
Prazosin	↓	→	↓
Prazosin+ propranolol	→	↓	→
Labetolol	→	→	→
Thiazides		↓	↑
Beta-stimulants	→	↑	→
Bendodiazepines		↓	
Phenytoin		↑	
Oestrogen		↑	↑
Progestogen		↓	
Alcohol 5 oz weekly		↑	
20 oz weekly	↓		↑

Key: ↑=increase; ↓=decrease; →=no change.

18

All forms of atherosclerosis are greater in diabetics but the reasons are not clear, nor is there any evidence that current therapy modifies the development or progression of this disease.

The diabetic diet may be a factor with the previously high fat diet in the UK and USA and low fat diet in Japan where, although the incidence increases in diabetics, coronary heart disease is still uncommon.

The role of hypertension and lipid abnormalities has not been shown to be a satisfactory explanation for diabetic coronary heart disease. It is most likely a combination of factors including obesity, hypertension, hyperlipidaemia, and increased platelet adhesiveness.[33] In the Whitehall study[34] the relative risk of coronary heart disease was doubled if the initial blood glucose was above 5.9 mmol/l (106 mg/100 ml) but with epidemiological data showing no lessening of risk for arterial disease even with improvement in glucose tolerance, the prospects for prevention do not encourage massive screening projects. However, the diabetic must be encouraged to avoid other risks, such as smoking etc.

Exercise

The role of exercise is one of the most conflicting.[35] It is difficult to differentiate the physical benefit from the psychological benefit of feeling fit. Studies have shown a higher

Table 2.5 Classification of hyperlipidaemias

Lipoprotein abnormality (increase)	Total cholesterol	Triglyceride	LDL-cholesterol	HDL-cholesterol	Lipoprotein phenotype	Clinical association
Chylomicrons	Normal to moderately elevated	Markedly elevated	Normal	Normal to decreased	Type I*	Acute abdomen pancreatitis
Low density lipoprotein (LDL)	Usually elevated, occasionally within normal range	Normal	Elevated	Normal to decreased	Type IIA*	Markedly increased risk of CAD
Low density lipoprotein (LDL); very low density lipoprotein (VLDL)	Elevated, occasionally marginally	Elevated	Elevated	Normal to decreased	Type IIB*	Increased risk of CAD
Intermediate density lipoprotein (IDL)	Elevated	Elevated	Normal to decreased	Normal to decreased	Type III*	Increased risk of CAD
Very low density lipoprotein (VLDL)	Normal to slightly elevated	Moderately to markedly elevated	Normal	Normal to decreased	Type IV*	Increased risk of CAD
Very low density lipoprotein (VLDL); chylomicrons	Slightly to moderately elevated	Markedly elevated	Normal	Normal to decreased	Type V*	Pancreatitis, increased risk of CAD
High density lipoprotein (HDL)	Normal to moderately elevated	Normal	Normal	Elevated	Hyperalpha-lipoproteinaemia	Decreased risk of CAD

*Fredrickson type.

19

mortality rate in bus drivers than bus conductors, post office sorters than delivery men but little change was noted in railway workers.[36]

The Framingham study showed only slight benefits for the active group of men and none for women. In Finland where physical activity is high, coronary risk is high, whereas Californian dockers, who indulge in high levels of physical activity, had a reduced incidence of coronary events, especially sudden death.[36] In a study of middle-aged civil servants regular vigorous exercise reduced the incidence of coronary events to a third of the sedentary, again with a reduction in fatal episodes.[37]

The benefit may relate to raised HDL levels and enhancement of the fibrinolytic response, but only in monkeys has exercise been shown to reduce atherosclerosis in those fed atherogenic diets.[38]

While the evidence for exercise as a beneficial occupation remains circumstantial, its role is probably significant when added to the principal risk factors. Combining the studies, a consistently favourable mortality benefit is seen with an average reduction of 20 per cent. Physical fitness in the presence of heavy smoking or other risk abuse, however, provides no protection.

Obesity

Obesity, in the absence of other risk factors, appears to be of minor importance.[39] Obesity, however, is frequently associated with other risk factors such as hypertension and diabetes. If obese people are more likely to have adverse lipid profiles, diabetes and hypertension, and consequently run a greater risk of developing CAD, they are relatively easy to identify and treat since this is frequently a familial problem.[40,41]

Personality and stress

In a study from Israel the lack of a wife's love and support coupled with anxiety proved to be as powerful a risk factor as cholesterol and hypertension with regard to coronary disease; the data from elsewhere are less conclusive and less sexist.[41,42]

Stress is a reaction by an individual in a non-specific way. It is incorrect to imply someone is 'under stress' if the assumption is that stress is some form of specific stimulus. Stress should be defined as an imbalance between the demands on an individual and the way the individual sees the demands. This is different for each person and generalized assessment becomes difficult.

Stress increases the heart rate, blood pressure, incidence of ventricular extrasystoles and raises the levels of catecholamines and free fatty acids. The secondary manifestations of stress can be modified by beta-blockade implicating the sympathetic nervous system.[43]

Certain environments may lead to stress. Men moving from rural to industrial areas increase their infarct rate three-fold. This may reflect social class pressure on the less skilled, since professional and managerial classes have shown a fall in coronary risk factors despite a consistency of lifestyle stresses. The figures may be distorted by non-stress factors, for example smoking cigarettes, which may be increased because of 'stress' on an apparently low stressed semi-skilled group.

Coronary events may be precipitated by stress and emotional trauma on a background of atheroma. Middle-aged widowers experience a death rate 40 per cent above that predicted in the six months after bereavement, and the prime cause is CAD. The cardiovascular death rate increased by 54 per cent in tea workers after the Bangladesh civil war of 1971 and by 50 per cent in a local population after the West Country floods in the UK in 1968. In the three weeks before infarction a significant increase in disturbing life events has been recorded, most beyond the control of the individual. There is, however, no evidence that these events provoke infarction in the absence of atheroma.[44]

Much has been made of personality types. Type A behaviour is competitive, aggressive, ambitious—life is full of deadlines, competition, impatience, and speech is explosive, gesturing frequently and the face taut and intense. The relaxed, 'laid-back' individual is designated type B. In the USA type A men have twice the risk for coronary heart disease than type B but in England type A civil servants have less than type B.[43–46] Type A behaviour is, however, not associated with the extent of coronary disease,[46] nor is there evidence that a specific link exists.

Given a background of summating risk factors, the presence of stress may act as a trigger when an artery is ripe for occlusion. In this context it represents a factor worthy of modification.

Alcohol

Alcohol taken in a limited amount appears to be of benefit.[47] Excess of alcohol may lead to cardiomyopathy and hypertension. Alcohol raises HDL as well as VLDL and the risk effect varies from individual to individual.

Although it may seem that wine confers an advantage,[48] it must be emphasized that alcohol susceptibility is variable, and women are more likely than men to develop higher blood levels for a given amount ingested. The advantage of wine is not shared by spirits or beer.

Coffee

The Boston collaborative study[49] implied that coffee could be harmful but this was not substantiated in prospective studies.[48] An additional study[50] suggests, however, that there is a dose-dependent/independent association between coronary disease and coffee consumption. Unfortunately an atherogenic diet could also be the explanation as this is more common in habitual coffee drinkers. Five or more cups a day appears to increase the risk

by two- to three-fold but these data are preliminary. Moderation would seem wise until further studies have clarified the situation.

Uric acid

Hyperuricaemia is associated with an increased risk of coronary heart disease but it is unclear whether this reflects associated problems (obesity, diabetes, hypercholesterolaemia) or whether it is an independent variable.[51] The Framingham study was not significant in men but of borderline significance in women.

Oral contraceptives

In the Royal College of General Practitioners Study, cardiovascular deaths increased five times for all women taking the contraceptive pill and ten times for those who had been on the pill for over ten years.[52] This risk is greater for women over forty years old, especially those who smoke cigarettes, have raised cholesterol levels, diabetes and hypertension.[53]

Contraceptives with progesterone as the major hormone lower HDL, whereas oestrogen-containing contraceptives have the opposite effect. Recently a dose-related adverse effect on blood pressure for the progestogenic part of the low dose contraceptive pills has been reported.[54]

Sex

There is no doubt that women suffer less atherosclerotic CAD than men. Only in diabetics is there no difference between the sexes. After the menopause the protection is lost with equalization of risk after ten to fifteen years.[55] It is tempting to attribute the difference to hormonal factors but significant lifestyle changes can confuse the issue.

In the Framingham study the premenopausal incidence of coronary heart disease was very low in those aged forty to forty-five years whereas those with an early menopause had a much higher incidence. This rise occurred after natural or surgical menopause but was unrelated to the removal of the ovaries.

Water

In the British Regional Heart Study[57] a negative relation existed between water hardness and coronary disease. The authors felt the association persisted after control for climate and socioeconomic factors with a 10–15 per cent excess in cardiovascular deaths in the areas with very soft water. The authors emphasize the absence of any physiological explanation, however, and duration of exposure needed either to induce or reverse an effect. No excess mortality was found in the thirteen towns with artificially softened water.

Paunches

Workers in Sweden[58] recently suggested that the size of the paunch in middle-aged men is a better predictor of coronary heart disease than other indices of obesity. While paunches were more common in coronary and stroke patients, so were hypertension and hypercholesterolaemia. Indeed, the sedentary may become flabby around the middle because of the inelasticity of abdominal muscle due to lack of exercise.

The paunch is a useful visible marker of a subject who may be at risk but it is not an independent factor.

Bad luck

For some, coronary heart disease presents in the absence of conventional risk factors. It strikes non-smoking, non-alcoholic, normotensive priests of the Catholic and non-Catholic faiths. There is no absolute protection!

Given the risks it is important to assess the proven benefits, and management is discussed in the next chapter.

PRACTICAL POINTS

- Risk factors are associated with disease and not definitely causative.

- Factors can be considered unavoidable (aging, male sex, diabetes) or avoidable (smoking, hypertension, obesity).

- The principle avoidable risk factors are cigarette smoking, hypertension and hyperlipidaemia.

- Possible factors which lead to a reduced risk include exercise, a cholesterol lower than 5.4 mmol/l (210 mg/100 ml), wine in moderation and a reduction in coffee consumption.

- Given the absence of a clear-cut cause for most of the population, a sensible lifestyle appears to be the most balanced option.

- Familial hypercholesterolaemia affects only 2 per cent of the population but with a substantially increased risk.

3
Primary prevention

BACKGROUND

Where possible prevention must remain the prime objective of all medical practitioners. Prevention can be divided into two groups:

- Primary (before the ischaemic event)
- Secondary (when evidence of ischaemia already exists).

Despite being able to identify the risk factors, primary prevention trials that aim to stop the development of the disease by modifying the risk factors have been disappointing overall. The principal risk factors as discussed earlier are cigarette smoking, hypertension and diet.[1]

SMOKING

Everyone is agreed on the need to stop smoking and to prevent the young from starting.[2] The benefits are obvious (see Figure 3.1) and it is rare to find people under fifty years of age with coronary disease who have never smoked. There remains a disturbing trend, however, among the young, especially women (see Table 3.1) who continue to smoke; perhaps this reflects the fact that in the UK the pro-smoking advertising budget was approximately twenty-five times greater than the antismoking budget in 1986. Over 70 per cent of smokers begin under the age of twenty, so it is obvious where education must be directed.

Antismoking literature should be available in schools. All schools should have lectures for pupils aged fourteen to fifteen or younger on the hazards of smoking, using simple graphics and vivid slides. Here family doctors, health visitors and community physicians have a major role to play.

Giving up

Most smokers want to give up and wish they had never started, yet only one-third succeed.

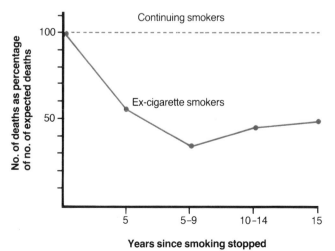

Figure 3.1 Reduction in coronary morbidity in men aged thirty to fifty-four years comparing smokers with those who stopped. (See also Figure 2.9.)

Doctors must clearly explain why the patient needs to stop smoking. Pictures and graphs to illustrate smoking-related diseases have a major impact. Another approach would be to tell patients to set aside a day, say the first of the month, and be prepared to experience discomfort and craving. These can be relieved by keeping busy, regular exercise and deep breathing. Reading, listening to music and the radio all helps. Patients should be advised to avoid environments where smoking occurs, such as parties, restaurants, the cinema. Weight gain can cause anxiety but it should be emphasized that giving up smoking is more important and excess weight can be treated at a later date. Snacks of fruit or low calorie biscuits can help if hunger is a problem. Patients must be prepared for irritability and boredom and may at first have a cough which seems worse than when they were smoking. They should be told that this is a good sign as it means the lungs are clearing themselves.

Help can come in different forms. Show them pictures representing death (see Figure 3.2); this may seem unduly dramatic but it has proved highly effective. Other options include nicotine chewing-gum, sugar-free mints or gum, acupuncture and hypnosis. In certain areas patients can attend groups to help them to stop smoking. Everyone is an individual, so it may be necessary to try a variety of remedies. If all else fails it is important to compromise. Patients should aim for three to five cigarettes a day, one after a meal and two others; any reduction, even if it is a very gradual one-a-day plan taking weeks, should be praised. A challenge from a team effort or raising money for the local hospital as a sponsored 'stop' gives a great deal of incentive. Switching to a pipe without inhaling can be a successful alternative.

DIET

Eating a prudent diet, increasing dynamic exercise and avoiding obesity sounds sensible but as a mass intervention there is little evidence to force a change in worldwide lifestyle.[3] Only those in the top quartile of serum cholesterol distribution[4] will actually benefit from lowering cholesterol levels. However, only one adequate study supports this philosophy: The Lipid Research Clinic Coronary Primary Prevention Trial[5] of cholestyramine. Studying the top 5 per cent of patients with raised cholesterol levels, those treated with the drug showed a 19 per cent reduction in coronary deaths and non-fatal infarcts. Confidence limits, however, were poor, making it difficult to extend the intervention argument to lower risk groups and from drugs to diet alone. There were non-significant reductions

Table 3.1 Smoking trends in the UK, showing an increase in the young and in women

Cigarette smokers (per cent)

	1977	1978	1979	1980	1981	1982	1983	1984	1985
All adults	39	37	38	39	37	35	34	35	34
All 15–19 years	30	30	29	29	29	30	30	30	31
Men 15–19 years	30	31	29	30	31	29	29	31	28
Women 15–19 years	30	29	30	28	28	30	31	30	33
Proportion of all smokers aged 15–19 years (per cent)									
	7	8	8	8	8	9	10	9	10

in the incidence of angina, abnormal exercise ECGs and referral for bypass surgery. This drug study, like all the others,[6-8] showed an increase in non-cardiovascular mortality with an increased incidence (often overlooked) of gastrointestinal cancer.

Advice

While the obese may benefit psychologically and physically from weight reduction, the important question revolves around specific dietary advice regarding a switch from saturated fats (palmitic and myristic) to polyunsaturated fats (linoleic) for those who are either overweight or at their optimal weight. From a philosophy of needing advice comes the need to screen the community and a realization that this advice implies a lifelong commitment to diet and possibly drugs. The risk is clear but the evidence is not strong enough for an obsessional change except in the very high risk group and even then drugs present anxieties, and diet must remain the primary method.

In general it is reasonable to adopt the 'little bit of what you fancy' approach in these circumstances. It is a fair compromise based on the evidence available. For those who are slim any diet must allow for adequate calorie replacement, and remember that diets deficient in red meat may lead to iron deficiency. Table 3.2 contains some practical guidelines. A shift from meat to fish and an increase in fruit and vegetables may be beneficial. When diet fails to reduce cholesterol levels in a high risk individual [cholesterol 6–6.5 mmol/l (231–250 mg/100 ml) age less than thirty years, 6.5–7.0 mmol/l (250–270 mg/100 ml) thirty to sixty years and 7.0–7.5 mmol/l (270–290 mg/100 ml) over sixty] drug treatment is the next option. This may not be such an important option in patients over sixty years of age but in the younger population the evidence is weighted to intervention. It may be worth a trial of fish oil capsules, which have been reported to reduce cholesterol by 27 per cent and triglycerides by 64 per cent.[9] However at present we have no indication of dosage needed, but side-effects are unlikely. The most effective drugs are cholestyramine with a 13–25 per cent reduction in cholesterol, probucol with a 10–27 per cent reduction, gemfibrozil with a 15–20 per cent reduction and bezafibrate with a 15–20 per cent reduction. All cause gastrointestinal side-effects and if these are a problem clofibrate should be tried, but only a 9 per cent reduction in cholesterol can be expected with this drug. Again gastrointestinal side-effects and possible increased malignancies can cause concern (Table 3.3). Bezafibrate is available in once-daily formulation, aiding compliance.

Individuals with high cholesterol levels should be given the following advice:

1 Lose weight
2 Change to a strict diet

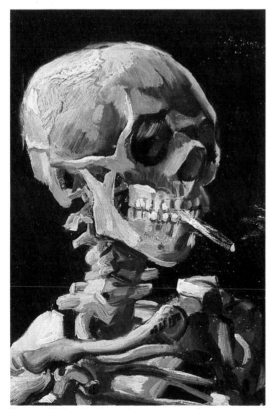

Figure 3.2 Making the message clear.

3 Increase exercise (and HDL)

4 Avoid drugs if possible

5 Keep all other risk factors under control

6 Take fish oil capsules but dose is unknown (? 5 g bid)

7 Drink wine in moderation

8 Advise friends of the new diet

9 Take probucol, gemfibrozil or bezafibrate after one year if still recording a high risk level of cholesterol (cholestyramine if tolerated)

10 Those with familial hypercholesterolaemia should be screened for coronary artery disease (CAD) by annual treadmill exercise ECG. Their relatives should be screened.

Table 3.2

Unrestricted foods
1 Chicken and turkey
2 White fish
3 Skimmed milk and cottage cheese
4 White of egg
5 Pure soya
6 Vegetable including pulses
7 Fruit — excluding avocado
8 Bread — wholemeal has highest fibre
9 Crispbreads
10 High fibre cereals

Foods which may be taken in reduced quantities
1 Lean meats — beef and lamb, pork and ham
2 Eggs — no more than two whole eggs weekly
3 Fat spreads — sunflower oil
4 Cooking oils — sunflower, safflower seed, olive oil

Foods best avoided
1 Fat and outer cuts of meat
2 Goose and duck
3 Offal — liver, kidney, tongue
4 Corned beef and luncheon meats
5 Sausage and paté
6 Shellfish and roes
7 All fried foods including crisps, etc
8 Dairy products — full cream milk, cream, hard and full–fat cheese, butter
9 Salad cream and mayonnaise
10 Malted drinks, cocoa, drinking chocolate
11 Biscuits, cakes, chocolate
12 Nuts

Hypertension

Controlling hypertension reduces the incidence of stroke, but the data for mild to moderate hypertension and coronary heart disease are not positive. The recent Medical Research Council (MRC) trial[10] of mild hypertension in the age range thirty-five to sixty-four years showed no benefit but 20–25 per cent of healthy men experienced side-effects from the drugs prescribed.

The European Working Party on Hypertension in the Elderly (EWPHE)[11] recruited subjects over sixty years of age with a diastolic pressure of 90–119 mmHg. They found a significant reduction in fatal myocardial infarcts from active treatment. Here we are dealing with older hearts with an increased chance of coronary disease. By reducing myocardial work as a result of reducing moderate as well as mild hypertension a benefit may be expected. Though a benefit from primary prevention on fatal infarcts is clearly possible, overall mortality was unchanged. This can be rationalized by a treatment plan, both non-drug and drug (if necessary), which should aim to reduce blood pressure in asymptomatic hypertensives over sixty years and thereby fatal myocardial infarcts. However, because overall mortality is unchanged, if drug side-effects are such that they ruin the quality of life, therapy could be justifiably withheld.

Given the benefits in reducing heart failure, renal failure and cerebrovascular disease, hypertension should, of course, be treated, but evidence of a primary preventive action on coronary disease is lacking. In the mild hypertensive subject based on the MRC data the first option should be drug-free with weight loss, perhaps a reduced salt intake, and modification of other risk factors such as smoking. If after a six months' trial the blood pressure remains raised, therapy should be instituted with low dose beta-blockade or a thiazide diuretic based on appropriate patient criteria. Side-effects should be carefully monitored to make sure that the quality of life remains acceptable. I most frequently use atenolol 50 mg at night to avoid daytime lethargy side-effects, or triamterene 50 mg plus hydrochlorothiazide 25 mg om.

Table 3.3 Profiles of currently available lipid-lowering drugs

	Clofibrate	Nicotinic acid
Indications	For primary dysbetalipoproteinaemia that does not respond adequately to diet. May be considered for the treatment of adult patients with very high (in excess of 8.5 mmol/l; 750 mg/100ml) serum triglyceride levels who do not respond to diet	Adjunctive therapy in patients with significant hyperlipidaemia (elevated cholesterol and/or triglycerides) who do not respond adequately to diet and weight loss
Total cholesterol-reducing efficacy	6.5–9 per cent reduction	9–10 per cent reduction
Compliance	Good	Poor
Most commonly reported adverse reactions	Most common is nausea; less frequent gastrointestinal reactions are vomiting, loose stools, dyspepsia, flatulence and abdominal distress	Severe flushing, abnormal liver function tests, jaundice, gastrointestinal disorders
Less commonly reported reactions but worth noting	Increased incidence of cholelithiasis. Flu-like symptoms. Increase in cardiac arrhythmias and intermittent claudication. Possible increased risk of malignancies	Activation of peptic ulcers. Decreased glucose tolerance. Hypotension. Increased cardiac arrhythmias
Known interaction with other drugs	Yes (anticoagulants)	Yes (antihypertensive drugs)
	Cholestyramine, colestipol	**Probucol**
Indications	Adjunctive therapy to diet for reduction of raised serum cholesterol in patients with primary hypercholesterolaemia (raised low density lipoproteins)	Reduction of raised serum cholesterol in patients with primary hypercholesterolaemia (raised low density lipoproteins) who have not responded adequately to diet, weight reduction and control of diabetes mellitus
Total cholesterol-reducing efficacy	13.4–25 per cent reduction	Ranges from 10.7 to 27 per cent reduction
Compliance	Poor	Good
Most commonly reported adverse reactions	Constipation, abdominal pain and distension, belching, flatulence, nausea, vomiting and diarrhoea	Most commonly affected is the gastrointestinal tract: diarrhoea, flatulence, abdominal pain, nausea and vomiting
Less commonly reported reactions but worth noting	Severe constipation. Increased bleeding tendency (due to vitamin K deficiency)	Slight prolongation of QT interval in some patients
Known interaction with other drugs	Yes (may bind other drugs given concomitantly, delaying or reducing their absorption)	The addition of clofibrate to probucol is not recommended
	Bezafibrate	**Gemfibrozil**
Indications	Hyperlipidaemias of type IIa, IIb, III, IV and V, which do not respond to diet alone	For dyslipidaemias which cannot be corrected by diet alone
Total cholesterol-reducing efficacy	15–20 per cent reduction	15–20 per cent reduction
Compliance	Good	Good
Most commonly reported adverse reactions	Most common are gastrointestinal effects such as dyspepsia. Skin rashes and pruritus	Abdominal pain, diarrhoea, nausea, epigastric pain, vomiting and flatulence
Less commonly reported reactions	Hair loss in men; very rarely myositis	Rash, dermatitis, pruritus urticaria, impotence, headache, dizziness, blurred vision, painful extremities and rarely myalgia accompanied by increases in creatine kinase
Known interactions with other drugs	Potentiation of anticoagulants. Additive cholesterol-lowering effect with guar gum; a similar effect may be anticipated with colestipol and cholestyramine although the doses should be taken several hours apart to avoid possible interaction of drug and resin	Anticoagulant dosage may require reduction

Screening

Two philosphies exist: mass intervention where each individual changes his lifestyle, and selective intervention concentrating on those at high risk.

A compulsory mass intervention would not work nor is there the scientific justification to enforce it. Advice at the mass level on cigarette smoking, sensible dietary habits and treatment of hypertension makes sense. Although there is still the practical difficulty of identifying cases at risk from a population who do not routinely go for medical checks, let us assume we are convinced of the value of treating hypercholesterolaemia. There are over 12 million men in the UK aged fifteen to sixty years and it would take a major effort and expense to check their cholesterol levels.

To concentrate on identifying the high risk individuals is also unrealistic because it is generally a group not obviously at risk and the entire population would need to be checked.

Selective screening of cholesterol in relatives of young infarcts, those with xanthomas or premature arcus (here opticians could be invaluable) is feasible. Everyone who visits the family doctor for whatever reason should have his blood pressure taken: 60 per cent of a practice will be covered in one year and 90 per cent in five years. A policy of annual blood pressure checks would not be difficult ('on your birthday each year'). The healthy could have their blood pressure checked by the dentist who sees individuals who are otherwise well and unlikely to visit the doctor. This would be cheap, simple and effective.

PRACTICAL POINTS

- Primary prevention attempts to prevent coronary disease before it starts.

- Only stopping smoking is proved to be of benefit to the general population.

- For those with familial hypercholesterolaemia diet plus cholestyramine is of proven cardiac benefit. However, no drug study has yet shown a reduction in *overall* mortality.

- In the asymptomatic hypertensive patient aged over sixty years, treating hypertension reduces fatal myocardial infarcts.

- Diet is important but other than familial hypercholesterolaemia there is no mandate for an obsessional change.

- A general commonsense approach is advocated with a diet avoiding excesses of animal fat, lubricated with a little wine, but not allowing obesity.

- Smoking should be avoided, ie, not started, and hypertension should be treated to avoid the risks other than those of CAD.

- Enjoyable exercise should be encouraged.

- To achieve primary prevention we need a major investment in educating the young.

4
Symptoms

BACKGROUND

Myocardial ischaemia, usually secondary to obstructive coronary artery disease (CAD), may present in several ways. Angina, myocardial infarction and sudden death are the most frequent clinical syndromes but heart failure and symptoms from arrhythmias are occasional primary presentations.

The diagnosis of angina or any form of heart disease has enormous implications not only for the patient but also for his family. Ischaemic heart disease threatens the well-being of the individual and his working, social, family and marital life. It is as much a psychosocial problem as a haemodynamic and prognostic one. It is therefore a diagnosis not to be made lightly and if there is a reasonable doubt this must be clarified. Above all the diagnosis depends on the accurate interpretation of the patient's symptoms. Unfortunately in the real world these may not be precise or clear-cut and when this occurs, a further opinion should be sought in the best interest of the patient.

CHEST PAIN

There are many causes of chest pain, secondary to disorders of the many structures within the chest. Clinically we are usually concerned with differentiating the pain of angina pectoris from chest wall pain, oesophageal pain, or functional pain perhaps linked to the hyperventilation syndrome.

Chest pain may be acute at the onset, usually within the previous few minutes or hours, or chronic, either present for days, weeks, or occasionally months. Pain for 'years' is usually not cardiac but exceptions do occur. Clearly an acute pain may be superimposed on a chronic history, eg, infarction on angina.

ANGINA

Angina pectoris is a clinical symptom sometimes supported by the ECG. A normal resting ECG does not rule out significant CAD.

Historical background

It was William Heberden (1710–1801)[1] who introduced the term 'angina pectoris' and there is little room for improvement in his classic description of its clinical effects, except to emphasize that shortness of breath is interpreted differently by individual patients and may represent a genuine symptom of angina.

'There is a disorder of the breast, marked with strong and peculiar symptoms, considerable for the kind of danger belonging to it, and not extremely rare, of which I do not recollect any mention among medical authors. The seat of it and sense of strangling and anxiety with which it is attended may make it not improperly be called Angina pectoris.

'Those who are afflicted with it, are seized while they are walking, and more particularly when they walk soon after eating, with a painful and most disagreeable sensation in the breast, which seems as if it would take their life away, if it were to increase or to continue: the moment they stand still, all this uneasiness vanishes. In all other respects the patients are at the beginning of this disorder perfectly well, and in particular have no shortness of breath, from which it is totally different'.

He did not, however, differentiate angina pectoris from cardiac infarction nor did he divide it into stable or unstable forms—yet so precise were his observations that unwittingly he records these variations as well as establishing the risk of sudden death.

'After it has continued some months, it will not cease so instantaneously upon standing still; and it will come on, not only when the persons are walking but when they are lying down and oblige them to rise up out of their beds every night for many months together . . . .

'When a fit of this sort comes on by walking, its duration is very short, as it goes off almost immediately upon stopping. If it comes on in the night, it will last an hour or two; and I have met with one, in whom it once continued for several days, during all which time the patient seemed to be in imminent danger of death.

'When I first took notice of this distemper, and could find no satisfaction from books, I consulted an able physician of long experience, who told me that he had known several ill of it and that all of them had died suddenly'.

Heberden goes on to describe the location of pain and its radiation and records its unpredictable pattern as well as 'the relief afforded by wine and spiritous cordiales'. He did not establish an aetiology but suggested a 'spasmodic disorder'. This does not mean coronary artery spasm nor is it possible that he thought of coronary spasm because at that time the relationship of disease of the coronary arteries to angina had not even been considered.

Heberden later reported a remarkable letter in response to his description, which he read at the College in November 1772.[2]

'. . . as well as I can recollect it is about five or six years since, that I first felt the disorder which you treat of; it always attacked me when walking, and always after dinner, or in the evening. I never once felt it in a morning, nor when sitting, nor in bed. The first symptom is a pretty full pain in my left arm a little above the elbow; and in perhaps half a minute it spreads across the left side of my breast and produces either a little faintness or a thickness in my breathing; at least I imagined so, but the pain generally obliges me to stop. At first . . . it went off instantaneously, but of late by degrees; and if, through impatience to wait its leaving me entirely, I resumed my walk, the pain returned . . . Sometimes I have felt it once a week, other times a fortnight, a month or a longer time may elapse without its once attacking me; but, I think I am more subject to it in the winter, than in the summer months'.

The author went on to describe sensations 'which seem to indicate a sudden death' which were probably secondary to an arrhythmia. Indeed sudden death befell the letter writer three weeks later and a post-morten examination carried out by Heberden and John Hunter again failed to take account of the coronary anatomy.

John Wall (1708–1776) and John Fothergill (1712–1780)[3] both described the angina syndrome and Fothergill along with Hunter noted at post-mortem examination in a typical case:

'The two coronary arteries, from their origin to many of their ramifications upon the heart, were become one piece of bone . . .'

and yet no concept of restricted supply down diseased coronary arteries was advocated. Edward Jenner (1749–1823)[4] in his letter to Heberden (1778) expresses concern that John Hunter has angina pectoris. Although he states his dissections throw little light on the cause of angina pectoris, he adds 'except that the coronary artery appeared thickened'. He then records a case when he found the same appearance of the coronary arteries 'with a considerable quantity of ossific matter dispersed irregularly'. He then wonders 'Is it possible this appearance may have been overlooked?'.

For the first time a connection is made between CAD and angina pectoris.

'The importance of the coronary arteries, and how much the heart must suffer from their not being able duly to perform their functions (we cannot be surprised at the painful spasms) is a subject I need not enlarge upon, therefore shall only just remark that it is possible that all the symptoms may arise from this one circumstance'.

Samuel Black,[5] a little known Irish physician, records similar findings in 1794 but it is left to Calib Hillier (James) Parry (1755–1822) to approach our current concepts of the mechanism for ischaemic pain.[6] As well as describing syncope and carotid sinus massage, he offers the following explanation for the ischaemic symptoms:

'though a heart so diseased may be fit for the purposes of common circulation, during a state of bodily and mental tranquillity, and if health otherwise good, yet when unusual exertion is required, its powers may fail, under the new and extraordinary demand .... It may not, indeed, be easy always to determine, by external marks, what degree of contraction can be termed excessive. That degree must certainly be relative to the heart itself'.

Nature of the pain
Ischaemic chest pain can be defined by asking the following questions:

1 Site—Where is the pain?
2 Radiation—Where does it go?
3 Character—What does the pain feel like?
4 Cause—What brings on the pain?
5 Relief—What do you do when you have the pain?

Site
This is usually retrosternal and can be surprisingly localized, but is more often across the chest. The patient may identify the pain by placing the flat of his hand across the chest

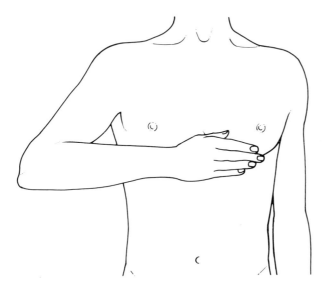

Figure 4.1 Patient may draw the flat of his hand across his chest.

(see Figure 4.1) or clenching his fist over the sternum (Levine's sign) (see Figure 4.2) as if to describe the squeezing and constriction sometimes felt. The patient can rarely localize the pain by pointing (see Figure 4.3). This is almost invariably musculoskeletal pain.

Radiation

The pain is referred to the neck or throat, leading to a choking sensation or constriction with perhaps a complaint of difficulty in swallowing (angina, from the Latin *angere*—to

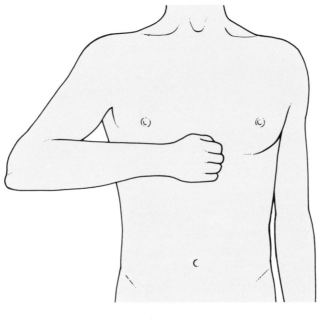

Figure 4.2 Clenched fist in the centre vividly illustrating the constriction or tightness felt.

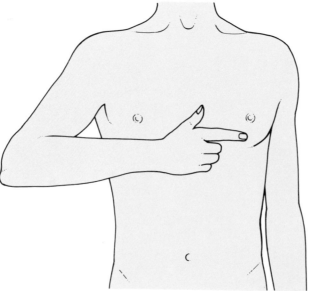

Figure 4.3 Almost never points to the pain as if localized.

strangle or suffocate). The latter may lead to the patient believing that he has indigestion, particularly when angina comes on after a heavy meal. Similarly radiation to the jaw (lower more than upper) can mislead the patient into thinking he has toothache or poorly fitting dentures.

Commonly the pain radiates to the left arm, occasionally the right or both arms. Cardiac pain usually passes down the inside of the arm under the axilla to the inner two fingers, whereas musculoskeletal pain is usually felt over the shoulder or outside the upper arm (see Figure 4.4).

Referral to the abdomen may imitate peptic ulcer pain or back pain suggest arthritis. Presentation in referral sites only is unusual (see Table 4.1) but can be dangerous, particularly

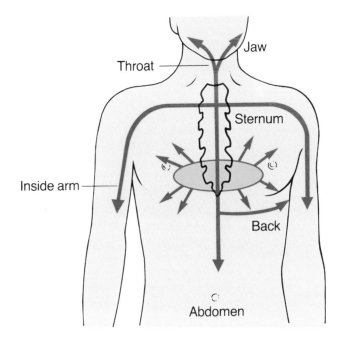

Figure 4.4 Site and radiation of cardiac pain.

Location of pain	Sole involvement per cent	Partial involvement per cent
Anterior chest	34.0	96.0
Left arm (upper)	0.7	30.7
Left arm (lower)	1.3	29.3
Right arm (upper)	0	10.0
Right arm (lower)	0	13.3
Back	0.7	16.7
Epigastrium	0.7	3.3
Forehead	0	6.0
Neck	2.0	22.0
Chin and perioral area	0	8.7

Table 4.1 Sites of anginal pain in 150 successive ambulatory patients

if there is severe epigastric pain which may even lead to a laparotomy. Usually there is an exertional or emotional component to help out, but for many the description of cardiac pain is vague and difficult to describe, and the pain does not fit into the convenient diagnostic box.

Pain usually radiates out from the chest rather than into the chest. I cannot remember a localized left chest pain 'in the nipple area' having a cardiac origin. It is possible, however, to have localized pain at the site of previous injury, eg, exertional pain involving a fractured arm, carious tooth or site of severe spondylosis.

Character (see Table 4.2)

The sensation may be so mild that it is almost dismissed by the patient—'its not a pain, more of an ache'. It is characterized by a tightness, a pressure, a heavy feeling, a constriction or frequently the tightness is perceived as a breathlessness. The pain usually builds up gradually over seconds or minutes rather than commencing instantaneously.

Table 4.2 Chest pain characteristics

Cardiac	Non-cardiac
Tightness	Sharp (not severe)
Pressure	Knife-like
Weight	Stabbing
Constriction	'Like a stitch'
Ache	'Like a needle'
Dull	Pricking feeling
Squeezing feeling	Shooting
Soreness	Reproduced by pressure or position
Crushing	Can walk around with it
'Like a band'	Continuous: 'It's there all day'
Breathless (tightness)	

Breathlessness as a symptom needs probing—'What do you mean by breathlessness, do you feel tight or just winded'—because far too many people are wrongly diagnosed as respiratory or heart failure cases instead of angina sufferers. A sharp, sudden, knife-like pain (often localized) is not cardiac. Local dialects need considering however; 'sharp' in south London means severe, not knife-like. Anginal pain tends to be constant while present. *Reader's Digest* pain, 'my heart is squeezed as if in a vice with a great weight on my chest' should be viewed circumspectly.

Watching the patient can be most helpful, particularly the way he moves his hand across the chest (see Figures 4.1–4.3).

Precipitating causes

Angina pectoris is brought on by an increase in oxygen demand that cannot be met by supply. The coronary arteries fill in diastole. With a supply and demand problem caused by obstructive CAD, any factor increasing heart rate (ie, demand) at the expense of supply (shorter diastole) can induce pain. Pain typically follows exertion, emotion (especially anxiety or anger), a large meal and temperature change. The pain is usually present on walking, especially uphill, is worse in cold or windy weather or after a meal if exercise is taken too soon. A meal can increase the cardiac workload by up to 20 per cent, a bath by up to 20 per cent. So a bath, a meal and walking the dog may induce pain more readily than at other times.

While for some the onset of angina is entirely predictable, for others there is considerable variation perhaps because of environmental or emotional factors. Exciting films or a vivid dream can induce pain, as can sexual intercourse, especially if the partner is extramarital or casual.

Stable angina of effort often leads to shop window gazing, stopping to chat or admiring the scenery to enable the pain to be rapidly relieved by rest.

Pain relief

A slowing of the heart rate by rest or relaxation will reduce demand. The patient may walk slowly, sit down or use glyceryl trinitrate sublingually. Pain relief is rapid, usually less than 10 minutes, and activity can then be resumed. Some patients relieve their pain by belching or taking antacids, which leads to the diagnosis of indigestion, but it is not the antacids that stop the pain but the action of stopping and resting while taking out the medication.

The trinitrin test, where the symptoms are relieved by sublingual nitrates, is unpredictable since often the nitrates relieve oesophageal spasm. Added to the other characteristics of cardiac pain, however, it is very useful particularly when pain easily relieved is no longer helped or becomes prolonged to over 30 minutes. At this point the angina should be considered unstable and a myocardial infarction needs to be excluded.

UNSTABLE ANGINA

This condition has many names including acute coronary insufficiency, the pre-infarction syndrome, intermediate coronary syndrome and crescendo angina.

It is characterized by new (usually one month or less) or worsening angina and/or angina at rest. Exercise tolerance may be suddenly and dramatically reduced. Although the pain occurs at rest it is still relieved quickly by sublingual nitrates, in contrast to the rest pain of infarction. It is a dangerous and volatile condition which, if untreated, may lead on to myocardial infarction or sudden death. By definition, there is no enzyme rise as in myocardial infarction but the ECG during pain may reveal significant ST segment depression (see Figure 4.5). It represents a medical emergency, necessitating hospital admission to a cardiac care unit where, hopefully, the condition can be stabilized and investigated further (see page 72).

VARIANT ANGINA

This is also known as Prinzmetal's angina. It is caused by spasm either superimposed on a

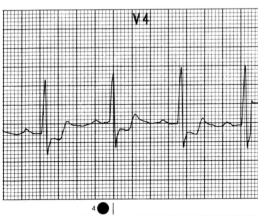

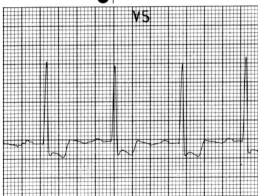

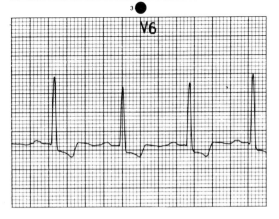

Figure 4.5 Unstable angina. Significant ST depression during pain.

fixed coronary lesion or in the presence of normal coronary arteries. It occurs principally at rest or in response to cold but may also occur on exertion (see Figure 4.6). In some it occurs at a consistent time of the day, usually in the night or early morning. In contrast with exertional stable angina, the patient frequently complains of palpitations at the time of the pain which in all other respects resembles that of classic angina pectoris.

The presence of ST elevation during the ischaemia separates it from the more usual ST depression of other forms of angina. It is promptly relieved by nitrates and calcium antagonists which reverse the vasospastic aetiology.

Other forms of angina

The ability to walk the pain off is unusual but well recognized, particularly if the exercise is pleasurable, eg, golf or hiking. This is known as second wind angina. Tobacco angina is rare but relates to pain at the time of smoking a cigarette or, more rarely, a cigar. Angina decubitus (pain worse in bed) is very unusual as an isolated phenomenon, patients almost always having daytime effort angina. It may be caused by dreams, a cold bedroom or cold sheets. The old teaching that it was syphilitic is now outmoded.

MYOCARDIAL INFARCTION

For some this is the first episode of chest pain; for some angina has been diagnosed before-

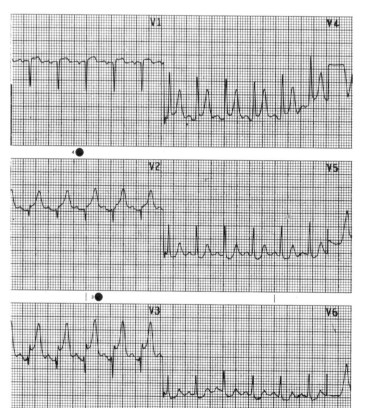

Figure 4.6 Variant angina. ST elevation in leads V1–V4 (a) and its reduction by sublingual nitrates in 2 minutes (b). The patient had a critical left anterior descending coronary lesion.

(a)

hand and for others the warning signs were dismissed as indigestion. Occasionally the onset is pain-free (the elderly, the diabetic, or a heart transplant recipient) or the pain is overridden by a complication such as severe breathlessness from acute pulmonary oedema. Infarction during general anaesthesia still occurs and may be missed completely.

The pain of infarction lasts longer than the pain of angina, and cardiac pain lasting longer than 30 minutes is infarction until proved otherwise. The pain is more severe, usually retrosternal, associated with pallor, perspiration—'did it make you sweat?—nausea or vomiting. Rarely inferior infarcts cause pericarditis which irritates the diaphragm causing hiccups. Radiation may occur as for angina or rarely the pain may occur in a radiation site only. It is not totally relieved by nitrates but may be modified.

Myocardial infarction may present via a complication. This is especially a problem in old people who may have an embolic stroke or show the signs of hypotension and shock. Anyone presenting for the first time with heart failure of no obvious cause should be investigated fully to exclude an acute myocardial infarction.

DIFFERENTIAL DIAGNOSIS

From the cardiac point of view there are two important differential diagnoses: acute pericarditis and dissecting aortic aneurysm. Non-

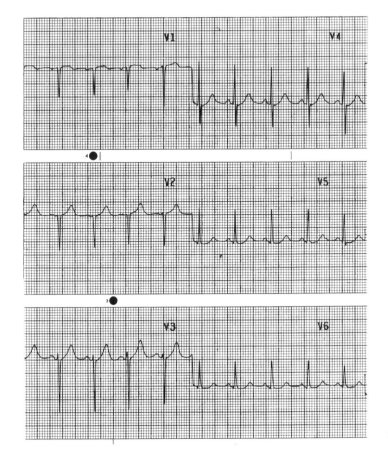

(b)

cardiac causes of chest pain include pain secondary to pulmonary disease, gastrointestinal problems, musculoskeletal pain, and functional chest pain.

Acute pericarditis

The pain from the rapid onset of pericarditis may be confused with angina though it usually has a pleuritic, sharp nature. It may increase with inspiration and when lying flat but be relieved by quiet shallow breathing or sitting up.

The pain may be constant and aggravated by positional change with referral to the abdomen. The pain of myocardial infarction does not vary with position. Because of the close relationship of the pleura the pain may be lateral and worse on coughing and it may radiate though the phrenic nerve to the neck and shoulder.

A pericardial friction rub confirms the diagnosis but in many this cannot be heard or is often transient. It is most frequently heard in the fourth left intercostal space with the patient leaning forward. Its characteristic is a dry scratchy sound out of step with the heart sounds. Pericarditis may be frequently associated with acute myocardial infarction but in the younger person an acute viral illness is the most likely cause. Pericarditis may complicate malignancy, especially bronchial, collagen disorders, renal failure or a primary cardiac tumour.

Late after infarction as part of a systemic illness (Dressler's syndrome, see page 111), pericarditis can be a troublesome relapsing problem.

Dissecting aortic aneurysm

Invariably a dissection leads to a very severe pain radiating to the back. Frequently the patient is shocked or a syncopal episode occurs. Radiation of the pain to the arms is rare unless the dissection has led to an occlusion of a coronary artery, when both infarction and dissection will coexist. Unlike infarction, the pain may radiate to the lower abdomen, thighs and hips. The pain is at its severest at its onset rather than building up as in infarction. Curiously patients often use the word 'tearing' to describe the pain of dissection, as if they know it is a tearing of the arterial wall.

Signs strongly supporting the diagnosis of dissection are: absent or diminished pulses, aortic incompetence possibly with pericarditis and, on x-ray examination, widening of the mediastinum. Neurologically, symptoms and signs will follow involvement of the cerebral vessels; renal failure secondary to renal artery involvement and ileus or diarrhoea reflect intestinal ischaemia. The pain is not affected by posture and the patient may have a history of hypertension. Early operation may save the patient's life and a rapid diagnosis is essential. The diagnosis should always be considered in those with poorly controlled hypertension, connective tissue disorders (especially Marfan's syndrome) and known coarctation of the aorta.

GASTROINTESTINAL PAIN

Oesophagitis

While oesophageal pain may mimic angina it rarely radiates to the left arm and it is not caused by exertion. It affects the patient when recumbent, especially at night, is worsened by bending over and can be exacerbated by a large meal. It can be relieved by belching, antacids, or sitting upright or standing.

The problem is that associated oesophageal spasm may be relieved by nitrates or calcium antagonists and with an incidence of reflux of 30 per cent in the general population it may easily be mistaken, diverting the diagnosis away from cardiac pain. Emphasizing the exertional component of angina pain usually resolves the issue.

A ruptured oesophagus is rare but the pain may be very severe, central chest radiating to the back. It follows vomiting whereas vomiting follows infarction.

Upper abdominal pain

A perforated ulcer with shock may imitate infarction or even cause infarction. The problem is usually that of a gastric diagnosis being made when the problem is cardiac due to acute epigastric pain (ie, referral site pain) without chest pain. An ECG should be done in all cases before surgery.

Acute cholecystitis may also cause confusion but tenderness in the right hypochondrium, nausea, colic and the absence of any exertional correlation beforehand usually clarifies the diagnosis. Chronic cholecystitis may have similarities with angina but again there is no exertional or emotional aetiology and there may be a history of intolerance to fatty or spicy foods.

Acute pancreatitis usually affects the epigastrium or back. It may be affected by positional change, relieved by leaning forward in a similar fashion to pericardial pain. The pain may be severe, the patient shocked and with signs of an acute abdomen. The serum amylase is usually raised.

MUSCULOSKELETAL PAIN

The number of people referred with clear-cut musculoskeletal pain is surprisingly large. While it is true that vertebral or costochondral pain can alarm the patient it is invariably localized, often positional and reproducible by localized pressure. This is a typical example of poor history taking and failure to examine the patient properly. Costochondral pain is not exertional but there may be tightness secondary to pectoral spasm. The patient may be breathless but this is invariably functional because of fear and hyperventilation. It is a frequent problem in young people under 'stress'. A simple careful history will elicit the diagnosis.

Localized vertebral pain is a little more alarming, suggesting the possibility of, and need to, exclude neoplasia.

There is no doubt that the failure to diagnose muscular pain delays treatment, induces neurosis and causes quite unnecessary referral to cardiac clinics.

PULMONARY PAIN

The pain from pulmonary emboli and infarction is usually pleuritic, associated with a cough and haemoptysis with worsening on deep inspiration.

A massive pulmonary embolus may be confused with myocardial infarction giving central chest pain, hypotension and shock. Signs or symptoms of a deep venous thrombosis, a recent operation or severe illness are helpful. The ECG does not show infarction, chest x-ray may be unhelpful, but the presence of shock without pulmonary oedema is highly suggestive of a large pulmonary embolus.

HERPES ZOSTER

Pain precedes the rash and the area involved is usually segmental. The diagnosis is confirmed by the appearance of vesicles on an erythematous base.

MITRAL VALVE PROLAPSE

This syndrome is associated with some typical, but usually many atypical, chest pains which are often recurrent. It is more common in women and the pain more frequent when fatigued rather than on exertion. The pain is often sharp anywhere in the chest, with radiation occurring very rarely. It may be brief or last for hours. Patients can usually walk around with the pain, which fails to benefit from nitrates. Palpitations are frequent. Clinically a mid to late systolic murmur may be audible at the apex, a click may precede it or a click may occur without a murmur. The click is often louder when the patient sits or stands. As a rule it should be thought of in the differential diagnosis of atypical chest pain in patients aged less than forty years, particularly in women with no obvious risk factors.

FUNCTIONAL CHEST PAIN

Pain in the inframammary region, left-sided, occurring more frequently in women and usually *after* exertion, is typical of functional pain. It may be very sharp or present all the time. It is often tender over the site of the pain.

Other names for this syndrome include effort syndrome, DaCosta's syndrome, neurocirculatory asthenia, and soldiers' heart. *Hyperventilation* is often a feature. Here air swallowing may cause gastric distension with pain inducing further hyperventilation as the patient attempts to relieve the discomfort. Chest wall tenderness and ache can follow overuse of the upper intercostal muscles and a substernal pain usually not related to exercise completes the picture. The pain of hyperventilation lasts for hours or days and is not exercise limiting. Other symptoms of hyperventilation include numbness and tingling of the extremities, light-headedness, giddiness and occasionally syncope. Patients may complain of a dry mouth and flatulence, sweating and excessive fatigue. They are often phobic with a fear of crowds, lifts or stuffy rooms. The respiratory features include difficulty taking deep breaths with the need to gasp or sigh at rest, undue and disproportionate dyspnoea on minimal effort, such as climbing two or three steps, and nocturnal breathlessness with panic.

Mixed pains

It follows that people who clearly have non-cardiac pain may also have angina and vice versa. Where doubt exists, and this is not uncommon, further investigations are needed to clarify the diagnosis and optimize management. There is no disgrace in writing as a diagnosis 'atypical pain but some typical features—not sure'.

BREATHLESSNESS

It is usual to associate the complaint of breathlessness with the respiratory system or heart failure. The patient, however, may feel the ache in the chest or tightness and constriction of angina as a form of breathlessness. When a patient says he is breathless the next question should always be 'What do you mean by breathlessness?' A surprising number mean tightness, with the obvious therapeutic implications being opposite to heart failure. If the patient does not clarify his symptom he must be led: 'Do you mean a tightness or panting for breath?' When both are a problem it is most often the tightness which comes first, pointing to the ischaemic angina aetiology. While studies have now shown that ischaemia can begin as pure breathlessness because of a rise of left atrial pressure, tightness and pain usually follows quickly.

Apart from hyperventilation the differentiation between cardiac and respiratory dyspnoea is not always straightforward, largely because both disease states often coexist.

Cardiac versus non-cardiac breathlessness

Here the diagnosis may need the help of a careful examination and chest x-ray. Cardiac breathlessness may be associated with murmurs, a gallop rhythm, raised venous pressure, evidence of pulmonary oedema (crackles and wheezes), hepatic congestion and peripheral oedema. The chest x-ray examination may reveal cardiomegaly and pulmonary congestion.

Acute breathlessness is the classic presentation of pulmonary oedema secondary to left heart failure. The patient may wake at night feeling the need for fresh air. He gets out of bed, coughs and wheezes and gulps in air. The usual variety is the need to stand up and is explained as going 'for a cup of tea'. The classic pink frothy sputum of pulmonary oedema is less frequently met. The relief of symptoms by walking about and going downstairs for a drink reflects the reduction in venous return secondary to positional change. Patients complain more of a persistent cough and night-time wheeze and relief from using more pillows rather than the more florid symptoms. The acute symptoms are frequently superimposed on a history of progressively decreasing exercise tolerance reflected in the New York Heart Association classification (NYHA) (see Table 4.3).

The clinical difficulty is separating an exacerbation of chronic obstructive airways disease from pulmonary oedema, since wheezes and crackles are frequently seen in both conditions.

Aside from the above, the respiratory patient may well have a preceding history of similar episodes. He may exhibit reduced chest movement, a pyrexia and localized signs of infection. Chest x-ray examination usually resolves the problem but in the presence of interstitial fibrosis it may be impossible to be sure and the only safe method is a trial of intravenous diuretics.

Table 4.3 Functional status according to NYHA

Class I

Patients with cardiac disease but with no limitation during ordinary physical activity

Class II

Slight limitations caused by cardiac disease. Activity such as walking causes dyspnoea

Class III

Marked limitation. Symptoms are provoked easily, eg walking on flat ground

Class IV

Breathless at rest

Similarly more than one condition can exist at the same time with the chronic bronchitic developing pulmonary oedema which then becomes infected. Since these patients are ill, therapy to cover all options (eg, antibiotics plus frusemide) is prudent.

Table 4.4 Some differential features of chest pain

Angina
See Table 4.3

Oesophageal
Not exertional. Rarely radiates to left arm. Worse when lying flat or after a large meal. Relieved by belching, standing, antacids but also by GTN and calcium antagonists

Pericarditis
Sharp pain worse on inspiration and lying flat. Relieved by shallow breathing and standing. Often pyrexial. Rub may be audible

Pulmonary
Pleuritic pain, worse with breathing, often localized. Frequent cough or haemoptysis. Rub audible

Musculoskeletal
Positional, localized, reproduced by pressure. Sharp, suddenly severe. May be tightness due to pectoral spasm. May be deep in the breast in women

Functional
Hyperventilation. Patient easily breathless, frequent sighs, anxious, often young woman. Musculoskeletal pain may be associated

Mitral valve prolapse
Mostly atypical but some typical pains and more common in younger women who may also hyperventilate. Frequently pain *after* exercise when fatigued

Dissecting aortic aneurysm
Very severe pain to the back. At its most severe at its onset. May radiate to the lower abdomen, thighs and hips. Not affected by posture

When a patient complains of chronic dyspnoea it is imperative to clarify what he means. A detailed history is essential but it must be remembered that many subjects are breathless on effort because they are sedentary, smokers and obese. Dyspnoea on effort, unlike chest pain on effort, may be benign. In women on the contraceptive pill when dyspnoea occurs with no obvious cause, multiple pulmonary emboli must be excluded.

PALPITATIONS

While chest pain can induce palpitations such as extrasystoles, or sinus tachycardia because of the pain or anxiety, the reverse, though well recognized, is unusual. In the elderly the onset of atrial fibrillation with a rapid ventricular response may induce angina for the first time, but it is pain associated with palpitations rather than palpitations alone which represents the ischaemic presentation. It is clear that if a patient complains of chest pain and palpitations it may simply be a matter of identifying the palpitations and treating them, leading in turn to a relief of the chest pain. This is a satisfactory option in the elderly but the need to exclude significant coronary disease remains essential in the younger population.

Table 4.4 lists the salient features to help in the differential diagnosis of chest pain.

PRACTICAL POINTS

- It is rare for the ischaemic patient to present silently.

- The diagnosis relies almost entirely on good history taking with the later support of technology.

- The diagnosis of ischaemia has important prognostic as well as psychosocial implications. It must be a definite diagnosis.

- If the symptoms are inconclusive do not label the patient without another opinion or confirmatory tests.

- Mild symptoms do not necessarily mean minimal disease.

- Tables 4.2 and 4.4 summarize chest pain features.

5
Stable angina pectoris—clinical evaluation

BACKGROUND

Obstructive coronary artery disease (CAD) is the commonest cause of angina pectoris. Other conditions with or without coexistent CAD should be considered in the diagnosis (see Table 5.1).

AETIOLOGY

In those over sixty years of age and occasionally in the younger patient, aortic stenosis and/or aortic incompetence need exclusion. In this situation it is important to auscultate carefully and be ready to seek a second opinion before starting therapy if unsure. Isolated systolic hypertension (systolic pressure > 160 mmHg, diastolic < 90 mmHg) may be a peripheral marker of aortic incompetence. With the increasingly elderly population, aortic valve disease is likely to be more frequently encountered, with important implications for detection and surgical correction.

Profound anaemia can cause pain in the absence of significant CAD by the combination of a reduction in oxygen availability combined with a tachycardia. It may also precipitate symptoms or aggravate a previously stable condition in those whose lesions may be mild or moderately severe.

Occasionally hypertension with left ventricular hypertrophy can lead to angina without coronary disease. There is usually an absence of other risk factors, such as cigarette smoking. Patients with sustained or paroxysmal tachyarrhythmias, especially atrial fibrillation in the elderly, or those with bradyarrhythmias usually secondary to sinus node disease, may also present with angina. Rarer primary causes of angina include hyperthyroidism, primary pulmonary hypertension and hypertrophic cardiomyopathy.

EXAMINATION

Usually no abnormality is found on examination. Inspection of the patient may reveal nicotine-stained fingers or the smell of tobacco. Anaemia should be excluded. Signs of hyperlipidaemia (see Table 5.2) include xanthomas on the hands, elbows, knees and ankles (see Figure 5.1); xanthelasma (see Figure 5.2) is surprisingly non-specific for hyperlipidaemia and arcus senilis, also non-specific in those over forty years of age (see

Table 5.1 Aetiology of angina

1 Obstructive CAD

2 Coronary spasm (usually rest pain)

3 Aortic stenosis

4 Aortic incompetence

5 Left ventricular hypertrophy (hypertension, cardiomyopathy)

6 Anaemia

7 Thyrotoxicosis

8 Rapid or slow arrhythmias

9 Severe mitral stenosis

10 Primary pulmonary hypertension

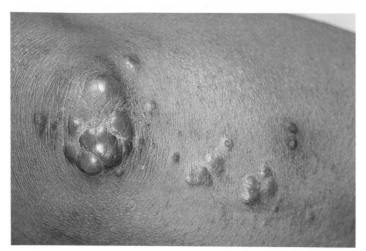

Figure 5.1 Xanthomas suggesting hypercholesterolaemia.

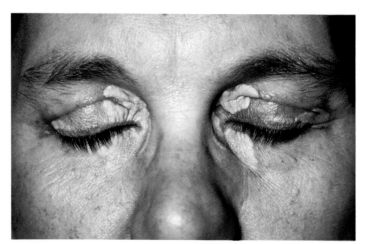

Figure 5.2 Xanthelasma. Non-specific sign.

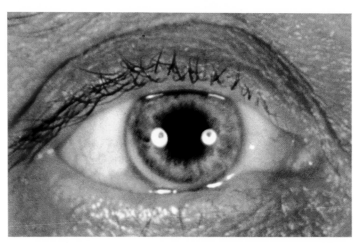

Figure 5.3 Arcus senilis. Non-specific over forty years but in the younger age group further evaluation is recommended.

Figure 5.3). The arcus may, however, be predictive in the younger age group and indicates a need for further evaluation.

The most frequent auscultatory finding is a IV heart sound (best heard with the bell of the stethoscope lightly placed on the apex), reflecting a reduction in ventricular compliance. Aortic stenosis and incompetence need to be excluded, and turning the patient on the left side may reveal a late systolic mitral murmur secondary to ischaemia of the supporting papillary muscles. Mitral stenosis presenting as angina is extremely rare and the patient will have other signs of advanced mitral valve disease with mitral facies because of a low cardiac output and a right ventricular heave secondary to pulmonary hypertension.

The cardiac impulse is usually normal but if felt during pain or after a previous, usually anterior, infarction a dyskinetic segment may be palpated. Extrasystoles may occur with or without pain and are relatively non-specific unless increasing during pain.

Hypertension may be present and signs of either carotid or peripheral arterial disease need to be looked for. Carotid or femoral bruits are the most frequent associated lesions but absent foot pulses, especially in heavy smokers or diabetics, may herald therapeutic difficulties.

A practical checklist is given in Table 5.2.

INVESTIGATIONS

These questions need to be answered:

1 Who is at risk?
2 How do we identify him?
3 Can we modify the risk?

The patient with severe symptoms in spite of optimal medical therapy has selected himself for further investigation with a view to surgical bypass. The decision here is simple. The main problem is to correlate mild symptoms

Table 5.2 Examination checklist

Sign	Location	Comment
Xanthoma	Hands, elbows, knees	Hyperlipidaemia
Xanthelasma	Eyelids	Non-specific
Arcus senilis	Eyes	Non-specific over forty years of age
IV heart sound	Apex (turn to left side)	Reduced ventricular compliance
Immediate diastolic murmur	3/4th left intercostal space, patient leaning forward	Aortic incompetence
Ejection systolic murmur	Apex, second right intercostal space, neck	Aortic stenosis
Late or pansystolic murmur	Apex to axilla	Mitral regurgitation
Bruits	Both carotid and femoral arteries	Peripheral arterial disease

with the extent of CAD. Unfortunately those with severe life-threatening disease may have minimal symptoms on medical therapy. A management plan is needed which will not only deal with the obvious but will also select those with a potentially avoidable catastrophic cardiac event.

Who is at risk?

Several studies have shown that prognosis is determined by the severity of CAD, particularly left main stem disease, and the extent of left ventricular dysfunction.[1] In order to judge the effect of medicine or surgery on prognosis, three major randomized trials have been conducted.[2-4]

The first trial, carried out by the Veterans Administration (VA) was conducted from 1970 to 1974.[2] At this time surgery was, in some centres, at a very early stage and the mortality rate of 5.8 per cent at thirty days

with only 69 per cent vein graft patency at one year reflects the lack of expertise. Because of this, the study has little relevance to current practice apart from recording the benefit from surgery for patients with left main stem disease in spite of the high operative mortality rate.

The other two studies which influence the investigation of the patient with angina are the European Coronary Surgery Study involving 768 men from 1973 to 1976 and the Coronary Artery Surgery Study (CASS) from 1975 to 1979, involving 780 American patients of whom seventy-four were women.[2,4] Important differences exist between these studies, with extremely important practical implications not only for identification of the disease but also modification of risk.

THE EUROPEAN CORONARY SURGERY STUDY This study was designed to ask the practical question of whether early surgery would improve prognosis in patients with mild to moderate angina pectoris. At five years 83.8 per cent of those randomized to medical treatment and 92.4 per cent randomized to surgery ($p < 0.001$) had survived. The operative mortality rate was 3.6 per cent, which is high compared with current rates— we now expect less than 2 per cent. Vein graft patency was 90 per cent at nine months and 77 per cent at eighteen months.

Medical therapy was poorly standardized but 74 per cent of patients were receiving beta-blockade. At five years 7.6 per cent of the surgical and 16.2 per cent of the medical group had died. This is a highly significant ($p = 0.00025$) 53 per cent reduction in mortality.

There was a significant five-year reduction in mortality for left main stem disease (see Figure 5.4) and in those with three vessel disease (> 50 per cent narrowing) treated surgically (6 per cent) compared with those treated medically (17.6 per cent, Figure 5.5).

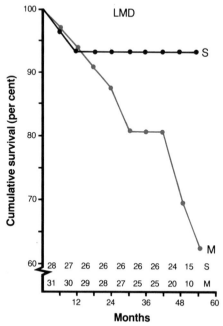

Figure 5.4 Improved survival five years after coronary bypass surgery in patients with left main stem disease (LMD). S=surgery; M=medical treatment.

Although there was no difference between medical and surgical treatment of patients with two-vessel disease as a whole, when one of the two vessels was the left anterior descending artery (LAD) with a stenosis before the first septal branch (ie, proximal) the mortality at five years was reduced by 60 per cent with surgery.

Those more likely to benefit surgically had an abnormal resting ECG and significant ST segment depression on exercise testing.

THE CASS STUDY This study excluded patients with left main disease and included those with either no angina or very minimal symptoms. It therefore did not attempt to answer the same questions as the European trial. Of 16 626 patients assessed only 780 entered the study indicating an unusual and very highly selected group of people.

At five years there was a 92 per cent chance of survival in the medical group and 95 per cent in the surgical group (not significant). Operative mortality was low: 1.4 per cent with graft patency at sixty days of 90 per cent. Only 43 per cent were taking beta-blockers.

No divisions into subgroups provided benefit at five years but after six years those with three-vessel disease and reduced left ventricular function fared significantly better if surgically treated (p < 0.01).[5]

RATIONALIZING THE TRIALS The European study investigated the management of patients with the symptoms of mild to moderate angina pectoris. The CASS study investigated patients with minimal or no symptoms.

The European study shows a clear benefit from surgery in those with symptoms, left main stem disease, three-vessel disease or two-vessel disease providing one lesion is in the proximal LAD. This study identifies a risk *and* a benefit. It is applicable to our current practice. It is all the more scientifically powerful when we consider that those who were in the medical group and had to have surgery for symptoms remained in the medical group, and that those assigned to surgery but who instead received medicine remained in the surgical group. If anything, the trial was weighted against surgery.

The CASS study states that people with minimal symptoms and a normal or only slightly abnormal exercise test with good functional ability and ventricular function can be safely followed medically.

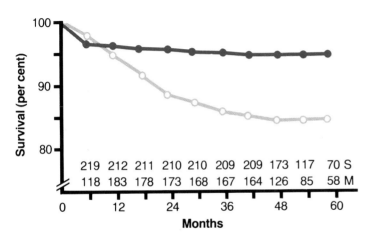

Figure 5.5 Improved five-year survival in patients with three-vessel coronary disease comparing medicine (M; ○———○) with surgery (S; ●———●).

Considering the prevalence of bypass operations per 100 000 population (see Figure 5.6) it is possible to appreciate that in Europe higher risk individuals are principally selected and operated on later than in the USA. The European and CASS studies support the correctness of this attitude regarding prognosis. However, financial limitations may be influencing judgment of what is a reasonable quality of life, and the low bypass rate may reflect the denial to significant numbers of people a more satisfying existence.

Identifying those at risk

In general practice the annual incidence of angina in men over forty years of age is five in 1000. In 75 per cent this is a primary presentation and in 25 per cent it follows a previous myocardial infarction. Each practitioner is therefore placed in an important front-line position for identifying the individual at risk.

General

The only absolute way of evaluating the existence and severity of CAD and left ventricular dysfunction is by angiography. Where practical, those below fifty years of age should routinely undergo this procedure. Because we are making decisions with prognostic implications for the next twenty to thirty years, maximum information is needed to provide optimal advice and treatment. Resources may not permit this philosophy and forty years of age may be the most practical arbitrary cut-off.

In patients over fifty (forty) years of age, treadmill exercise testing using a twelve-lead ECG system is an important and useful means of screening for at-risk patients with chest pain.

Specific

1 SCREENING   When asymptomatic subjects were screened with resting and exercise electrocardiography, a high incidence of false positive tests for CAD occurred.[6] Of 100 people having angiography two-thirds had normal coronary arteries. The routine use of screening exercise ECGs in an asymptomatic population was therefore not recommended. However, certain subjects may benefit from this approach, always with the proviso that many will subsequently undergo unnecessary angiography. About 2 per cent of the population in the UK have an inherited hypercholes-

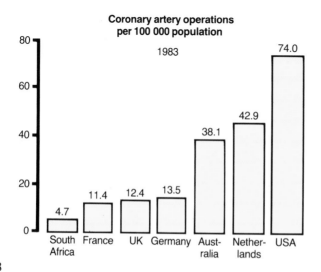

Figure 5.6   Prevalance of coronary bypass operations in seven countries. Note the low UK rate compared with Australia.

terolaemia and a case can be made for annual screening by exercise testing with, of course, a thorough check on close blood-relatives. It is fashionable for executives, members of parliament, doctors and various other professional groups to undergo treadmill testing as part of 'an executive screen'. There is always the danger of hypochondriasis after a positive test while waiting for the definitive normal coronary angiogram. The benefit is the reassurance of the normal exercise test or the identification of unsuspected CAD. However, from the CASS study we should only be operating on an asymptomatic minority who might have left main stem disease. The logic of prognostically screening asymptomatic people therefore relies solely on the belief that left main stem disease will be detected and lead to possible surgery. As left main disease represents only 8 per cent of the chest pain population and substantially less of the non-chest pain population, this argument has little substance or practical importance. The Civil Aviation Authority has rejected exercise electrocardiography for asymptomatic pilots.

2 ELECTROCARDIOGRAPHY *(a) At rest* A normal resting twelve-lead ECG does not rule out significant CAD in patients suffering from chest pain. An ECG during pain may reveal significant ST segment abnormalities, defined as 1 mm or more of horizontal or downsloping ST depression (see Figure 5.7). Similarly, ST elevation during pain points to variant angina (see page 77).

The resting ECG, however, is only helpful if it is abnormal, which is less than 50 per cent of the time.
(b) On exercise The treadmill exercise twelve-lead ECG is a safe and accurate noninvasive test for risk evaluation of patients with chest pain. Medical supervision is essential, for though the risks are few the consequences can be fatal. The mortality rate is 1:10 000 tests and the non-fatal complication rate 2.4:10 000.[7,8] The incidence of ventricular

fibrillation is 1:5000. Thus full resuscitation facilities should be at hand.

It is dangerous to exercise patients with:

- Unstable angina pectoris
- Significant aortic stenosis
- Pulmonary hypertension
- Severe systemic hypertension
- Known, poorly controlled serious ventricular arrhythmias.

However, in evaluating the patient with stable angina pectoris these exclusions very rarely apply.

The most accepted and acceptable test is the treadmill exercise ECG. It is most accurate if maximal and symptom limited. The Bruce protocol is the most widely used diagnostic test, providing an intense workload by progressive increases in slope and speed (see Table 5.3). The Naughton protocol is less intense and more applicable to high risk patients or those with skeletal mobility problems.

The main end-points for ischaemia are:

- Significant ST segment depression greater than 1 mm (see Figure 5.8)
- Slow ST recovery to normal
- Fall in systolic blood pressure (reflecting a fall in cardiac output)
- Angina at a low workload
- Dangerous arrhythmias such as ventricular tachycardia.

ST depression can be caused by digoxin, and beta-blockers may prevent its occurrence. Digoxin should be discontinued for 7 days and beta-blockers for 48 hours before the test. Nitrates and calcium antagonists seldom interfere with the diagnostic accuracy but if doubts exist the test needs repeating after they have been discontinued.

A rise in diastolic blood pressure by 15 mmHg or greater has been shown recently to point to significant coronary disease.[9] The mechanism is reflex vasoconstriction secondary to an ischaemia-induced fall in cardiac

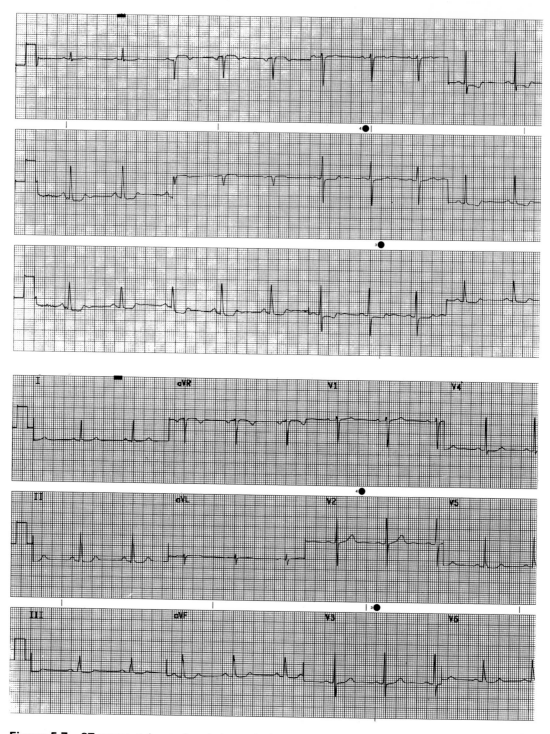

Figure 5.7 ST segment depression during pain (top trace) and after pain relief (bottom trace).

output which may precede ST change. Patients who become unsteady or fatigued, or show severe systolic hypertension, should have the test terminated. The development of greater than 3 mm ST depression without symptoms and before maximal exercise has been achieved also represents an indication for stopping the test—there is nothing more to prove.

The following exercise terminology is used:

True positive = positive exercise test/CAD

True negative = negative exercise test/ normal coronary arteries

False positive = positive exercise test/normal arteries

False negative = negative exercise test/ CAD

$$\text{Sensitivity} = \frac{\text{true positives}}{\text{true positives} + \text{false negatives}}$$
$\times$ 100 per cent

ie, the ratio of correct abnormal ECGs to the total number of angiographically abnormal cases

Table 5.3 The Bruce Protocol

Stage	Time minutes	Grade per cent	Speed mph	Energy cost METs
1	0–3	10	1.7	5.1
2	3–6	12	2.5	7.1
3	6–9	14	3.4	10.0
4	9–12	16	4.2	14.0
5	12–15	18	5.0	15.7

A MET (metabolic equivalent) is the resting oxygen consumption, usually 3.5 ml/kg per minute. The average individual of non-athletic status should be able to manage 10 METs.

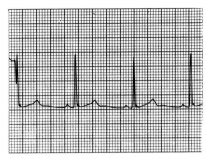

ECG at rest

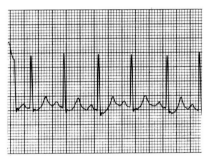

After exercise for 3 minutes

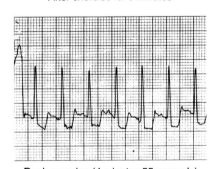

Peak exercise (4 minutes 55 seconds)

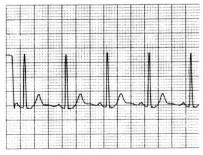

1 minute after exercise

Figure 5.8 Exercise ECG reveals significant ST depression indicating CAD.

51

$$\text{Specificity} = \frac{\text{true negatives}}{\text{true negatives} + \text{false positives}}$$
$\times 100$ per cent

ie, the ratio of correct normal ECGs to the total number of angiographically normal patients.

$$\text{Predictive accuracy} = \frac{\text{true positives}}{\text{true positives} + \text{false positives}}$$
$\times 100$ per cent

ie, the percentage of abnormal results that are true.

In patients with chest pain, exercise testing has a specificity for CAD of the order of 85 per cent and a sensitivity of 85 per cent. This means that it will fail to identify 15 per cent of patients with disease (false negatives) and indicate disease where there is not in 15 per cent (false positives). In other words, 15 per cent of those needing angiography will not get it and 15 per cent of those who do not need it will. Thus, on balance, treadmill ECGs miss few patients who are at risk.

NUCLEAR IMAGING Nuclear scanning has a limited, but helpful, role in addition to exercise electrocardiography. Immediate limitations are availability and expense in comparison with treadmill electrocardiography. It is, however, particularly useful when the resting ECG has characteristics which make it difficult to evaluate on exercise, especially left bundle branch block. It is also helpful when the patient cannot exercise well for various reasons such as arthritis, claudication or obstructive airways disease, or when the routine exercise ECG gives non-diagnostic or borderline information in a patient with an atypical story.

The commonest used tests are radionuclide ventriculography and thallium scintigraphy. Radionuclide ventriculography with Technetium-99 blood pool labelling measures ventricular function.[10] This is of value at rest and on exercise. It has a very important role in risk assessment after myocardial infarction;

furthermore, by monitoring exercise-induced left ventricular dysfunction, a sensitivity rate as high as 90 per cent has been recorded for ischaemia.

Thallium-201 is taken up by the perfused myocardium. Thus infarcted areas will be delineated as 'cold' areas failing to fill in. Exercise may identify cold areas which reperfuse later, pointing to reversible ischaemia (see Figure 5.9). Partial filling suggests ischaemia adjacent to an infarct. Specificity is of the order of 90 per cent and sensitivity 80 per cent.[11]

At present in patients with angina, twelve-lead treadmill testing is the cheapest most available and reliable noninvasive approach with nuclear scanning, of use in important subsets or when diagnostic doubts exist.

CORONARY ANGIOGRAPHY This specialist technique requires a day or two in hospital. Though it is a quick procedure (20–30 minutes) with minimal risk (1:2000 death rate)[12] it is expensive. With the patient under local anaesthetic, catheters are advanced from the femoral artery (Judkin's technique) or brachial artery (Sones' technique). Contrast medium is injected into the coronary arteries in multiple views using hand injections and into the left ventricle under greater pressure via a pump. The patient experiences a warm sensation for 90 seconds after the left ventricular angiogram. A small number of patients have a sensation of nausea or vomit after the first injection of contrast. This settles quickly.

Coronary angiography accurately assesses the anatomy of the individual coronary arteries and their branches and the left ventriculogram identifies areas of dysfunction which will influence management. A reduction in coronary arterial cross-sectional area of 70 per cent or more is considered to be important. The left coronary artery arises as the left main coronary artery, dividing into the LAD with its diagonal branches, and circumflex with its marginal or lateral branches (see Figure 5.10).

52

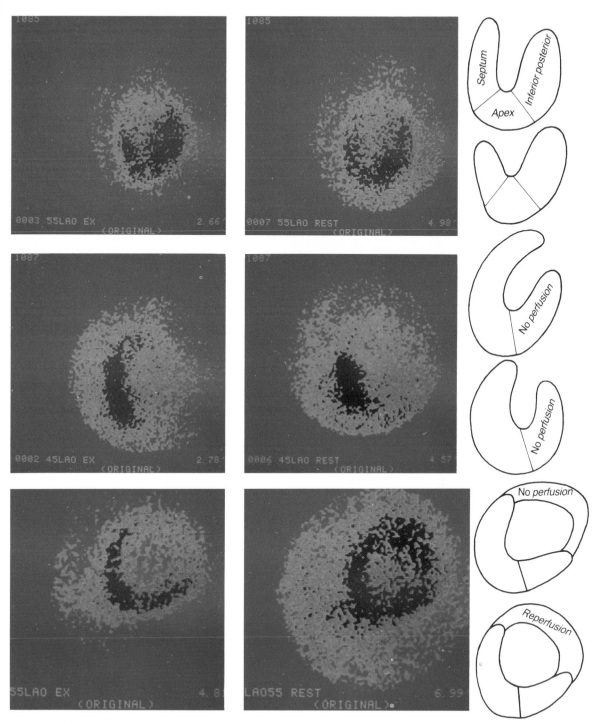

Figure 5.9 Thallium scintigraphy. (Top) Normal. Perfusion is complete at rest and after exercise. (Middle) Infarction. A deficit is seen on exercise with no reperfusion on resting. (Bottom) Ischaemia. Deficit on exercise with reperfusion after resting.

The right coronary artery continues into the posterior descending vessel from the crux. Depending on disease location in the three major vessels comes the terminology single, double or triple vessel disease (not including left main).

Left ventricular function is expressed in terms of the amount of blood ejected with systole—the ejection fraction (normally over 50 per cent) and areas of wall dysfunction (see Figure 5.11). These can be defined as hypokinetic (reduced movement), akinetic (no movement), and dyskinetic (paradoxical movement). A series of representative angio-

grams is shown in Figures 5.12–5.15. Angiography should be available to everyone whose symptoms interfere with their enjoyment of life, no matter how old, providing their general health is good. Those with abnormal ECGs on exercise, independent of the severity of symptoms, need angiography for prognostic reasons, and because prognosis is a function of the extent of coronary disease and left ventricular damage, all younger people should undergo diagnostic angiography to optimize the management for the many years to come.

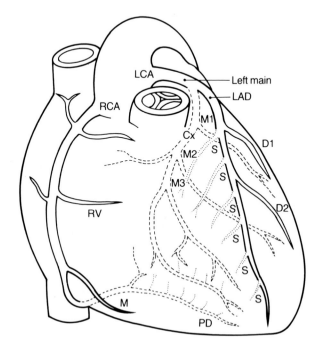

Figure 5.10 Schematic chart of the major coronary arteries. The posterior descending (PD) may arise from the right coronary artery (RCA; R dominant) or circumflex (Cx; L dominant). D=Diagonal; LAD=left anterior descending; LCA=left coronary artery; M=marginal branches; RV=branch to the right ventricle; S=septal branch.

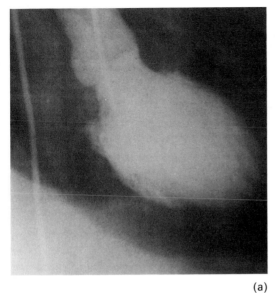

(a)

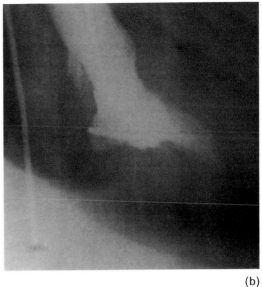

(b)

Figure 5.11 Right anterior oblique schematic
of left ventricular angiogram with normal still
frames (a) in diastole and (b) in systole. By
tracing these and subtracting, the percentage of
the blood ejected (ejection fraction) can be
calculated.

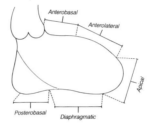

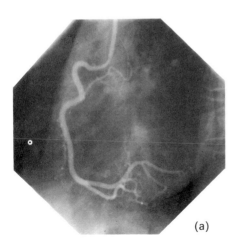

(a)

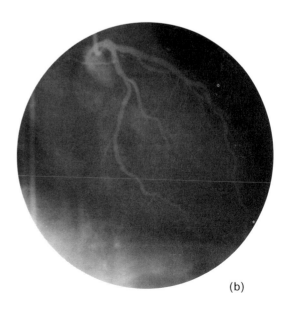

(b)

Figure 5.12 Normal right (a) and left
coronary artery (b).

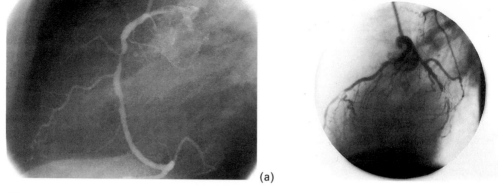

Figure 5.13   (a) Critical right coronary artery stenosis and (b) LAD and circumflex stenoses.

Figure 5.14   Left main stenosis.

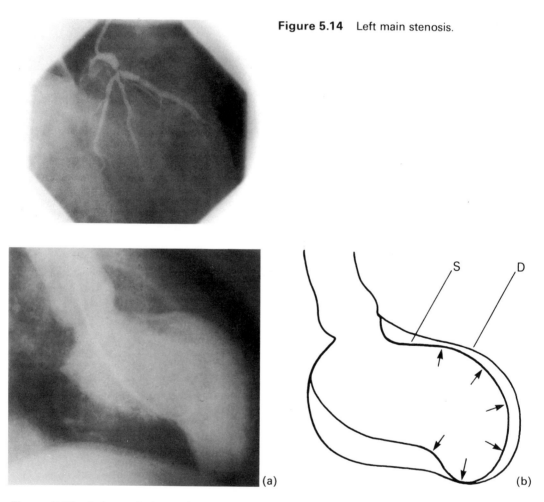

Figure 5.15   Left ventricular angiogram (systolic frame S) revealing extensive infarction in the anteroapical segment with the dyskinetic area D marked in small arrows.

Modifying the risk

The patient brings his symptoms; his quality and quantity of life rest in the hands of his practitioner. The summary chart (Figure 5.16) is designed to help with management decisions and referrals.

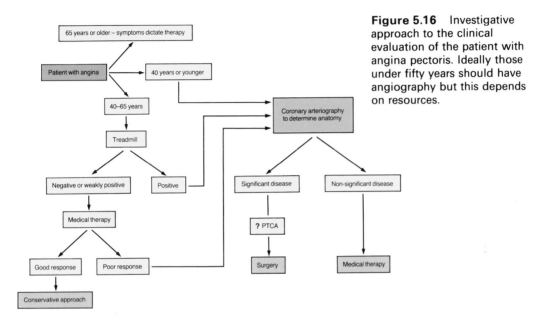

Figure 5.16 Investigative approach to the clinical evaluation of the patient with angina pectoris. Ideally those under fifty years should have angiography but this depends on resources.

PRACTICAL POINTS

- The main cause of angina is obstructive CAD.

- A good clinical examination may identify other causes, eg, aortic valve disease.

- Those under 65 years should have their risks assessed by exercise testing.

- The younger patient, under 50 years, should undergo detailed evaluation including angiography to optimize management for the next 20–30 years.

- Mild symptoms may hide critical disease. It is too easy to be complacent when there is a good response to medical therapy.

- Prognosis is related to the extent and severity of CAD and the quality of left ventricular function.

- Old people who are otherwise well but fail to respond to medical therapy should be offered further investigations. Age alone should not be a barrier.

6
Stable angina pectoris—management

BACKGROUND

The management of angina pectoris must take into account both the quality and quantity of life of the patient. It is not usually difficult to treat the pain but there is much more than just relief of symptoms.

PREVENTION

General advice

There is no substitute for a careful, clear explanation of the nature of the problem, the reasons it occurred and how the patient can help himself by modifying his risk status. It is important from the start to emphasize the team approach. Patients are often devastated by the diagnosis of a heart condition and time spent with them and their spouses is invaluable in putting the problems in perspective and guiding them forward positively. Booklets are available to reinforce the advice and to answer questions often forgotten at the interview, and these should be used routinely.

Patients must not be punished or instilled with guilt. Doctors must concentrate on reducing smoking which is responsible for 25 per cent of coronary deaths in those under sixty-five years and 80 per cent of men below forty-five. Cigarettes increase the myocardial workload by catecholamine stimulation at the same time as reducing oxygen supply by carbon monoxide inhalation (see Chapter 2, page 12).

Obesity increases the workload of the heart, and weight reduction can help to control pain. Doctors and dietitians should routinely advise on diet (see Chapter 3, page 24). All non-smokers under sixty-five, and all patients under fifty years of age, should have their lipid profiles checked for inherited hyperlipidaemia, which might identify a family at risk.

Regular exercise may improve the patient's well-being. While there is no statistical evidence that regular exercise reduces morbidity or mortality, studies show a consistently favourable trend. It is important to emphasize the need to enjoy exercise; there is no point advising patients to jog if they hate it, and it would be better for them to walk in the countryside. Isometric exercise (press-ups, weight training) should be avoided because of excessive heart rate and blood pressure rises. The advantages of a treadmill ECG in assessing risk and the need for investigations have already been mentioned, but a further usefulness is in giving the patient confidence in what he can do as well as guiding the practitioner or advising on the patient's physical abilities. For example, a patient with mild angina and a good treadmill response can safely go skiing.

Most people can maintain their employment, but heavy goods vehicle licences must be surrendered. Driving otherwise is permitted. Stress is a problem in the presence of other risk factors but not as an isolated entity. It is worth advising the patient to consider the emotionally demanding aspects of his lifestyle in the working and home environment. Regular holidays, non-stressful lunch time and home activities (gardening, reading) help complete the lifestyle change, which is usually easier for the patient to follow than expected.

Type A individuals may be more at risk than the relaxed type B counterparts (see Chapter 2, page 20). Here it is of interest that beta-blockade can induce personality change from A to B which may be useful in the appropriate patients with anginal pain.[1]

A question seldom asked concerns sexual activity. Stress on the heart during sexual intercourse is no greater than during normal daily activity providing the couples are married or have been cohabiting for some time. The casual relationship with its greater stress factor does lead to a more vigorous cardiovascular response. A useful practical guide is the rule of two flights of stairs: if the patient can briskly climb up and down two flights of stairs without symptoms, sexual intercourse will generally be angina-free. Extramarital sex is associated with a greater chance of a cardiac event, but may be preventable by drug therapy with nitrates and beta-blockade.[2]

DRUG THERAPY

Nitrates

Nitrates are potent venodilators and to a lesser extent arterial dilators (see Table 6.1). They alleviate the symptoms of angina by lowering the workload of the heart secondary to vasodilatation. Coronary vasodilatation occurs to a variable extent but peripheral effects are responsible for the majority of the benefit. Nitrates can be used safely and effectively in addition to beta-blockade and calcium antagonists.

Sublingual glyceryl trinitrate (GTN) avoids hepatic metabolism, is effective in 2 to 3 minutes and may be repeated. It may be used for the relief of angina or prophylactically. Glyceryl trinitrate loses its potency after two to three months and, if possible, should be

Table 6.1 Nitrate preparations

Preparation	Use	Comments
Sublingual GTN	Alleviates attacks quickly; prophylaxis 30 minutes	Headaches. Replenish every two to three months. Careful storage
GTN spray 400 µg	Alleviates attacks quickly; prophylaxis 30 minutes	Expensive. Headaches. Inflammable
Topical nitrates	Nocturnal symptoms? Debatable whether it is useful	Expensive, short duration of action, patch cosmetically better than paste. Tolerance + +
Isosorbide dinitrate 1 sublingual 2 oral	Prophylaxis 1 hour Prevention of pain. 10–40 mg bid	As GTN Hepatic metabolism + Tolerance + if tds or qds
Isosorbide mononitrate	Prevention of pain. 10–40 mg bid	Early results encouraging. 100 per cent bioavailability
Buccal nitrates	Alleviate pain and prophylaxis	Expensive, not well tolerated

stored in a darkened glass bottle in a fridge, without cotton wool. Glyceryl trinitrate spray delivers 400 µg with each jet spray, lasts up to three years but is more expensive. However it may be advantageous when the patient's pain is infrequent. The principal side-effect is headaches, about which all patients should be warned. Glyceryl trinitrate lasts up to 30 minutes sublingually and for a more prolonged effect sublingual isosorbide dinitrate may be preferred (eg, 5 mg before sexual intercourse).

Oral nitrates have until recently relied on hepatic metabolism converting the dinitrate to its active metabolite, the mononitrate. This has led to substantial variability in effect from patient to patient and between products, especially the slow release formulations. In addition, tolerance (decreased effect with time) has been reported within days.[3] The development of isosorbide mononitrate offers 100 per cent bioavailability and the early clinical trials are encouraging concerning its effectiveness and lack of tolerance.[4] Nitrate tolerance is probably caused by consistent (even) blood levels over 24 hours and mononitrate given bid avoids this. Slow-release formulations, maintaining an even 24-hour nitrate level, will be subjet to tolerance and should be avoided. Our current recommendation is isosorbide mononitrate 10 mg bid increasing to 20 mg bid and occasionally 40 mg bid. Based on the bioavailability data there is no longer the need for dinitrate preparations.

Buccal glyceryl trinitrate offers the advantage of immediate release of nitrate, though slower than GTN, with a more gradual release over 4 hours or so. It appears to be effective, variably tolerated, but expensive. It may be of value when oral medication is not possible as in the pre-operative or post-operative state.

Topical nitrates were developed to avoid hepatic metabolism and provide more consistent antianginal effects but unfortunately tolerance develops rapidly. This again is due to even blood levels throughout the day. In-

termittent use (12 hours on, 12 hours off) may be effective but is an expensive option.[5] They are mainly of value for nocturnal pain or breathlessness not responding to oral therapy.

Occasionally, as well as headaches, nitrates can cause postural hypotension though this is more common in the elderly. Overall they are the safest of all antianginal preparations and can be used in heart failure where a haemodynamic benefit may also be achieved (see page 155).

Beta-blockade

Beta-adrenergic blockade reduces sympathetically-mediated increases in heart rate, systolic blood pressure and myocardial contractility, thereby reducing myocardial demand. These actions, produced by competition at the beta-adrenergic receptors, lead to a reduction in angina attacks and need for GTN as well as an increase in exercise tolerance with less ischaemia on the ECG. Furthermore, the number of ischaemic episodes over 24 hours, whether silent or not, is reduced.[6,7] Beta-blockade is effective in over 90 per cent of patients.

In Table 6.2 the individual agents and properties are summarized. Some are *cardioselective* in that they preferentially block beta-one receptors in the heart rather than beta-two in the lungs or blood vessels. These are less likely to produce problems by blocking sympathetically-mediated bronchodilation and peripheral vasodilation as well as being less likely to impair glucose release in response to hypoglycaemia. They will, however, mask the tachycardia diabetics may be using as a warning sign. Selectivity is *relative* and decreases with increasing dosage of each agent, ie, atenolol 100 mg is less selective than atenolol 50 mg. Where doubt exists a calcium antagonist should be chosen.

Some agents, eg, pindolol or acebutolol have partial agonist activity and are theoretically less likely to produce extremes of bradycardia, bronchoconstriction or vasoconstriction. This is also known as intrinsic sympathomimetic activity (ISA). In patients with severe angina this may be a disadvantage because of lack of effect on the resting heart rate, whereas in those with peripheral side-effects the less depressant effect on cardiac output may substantially reduce the problems of coldness and heaviness of the limbs.

In general, beta-blockers are well tolerated and remain first-line drugs in the treatment of angina pectoris. Beta-blockade is competitive and the major reason for a poor response remains a failure to give enough medication. Because of the varying potencies of individual beta-blockers, it is important to be thoroughly familiar with the use of one or two agents (see Table 6.2). The resting heart rate is an unreliable means of determining the degree of beta-blockade and heart rates in the forties and fifties per minute that are well tolerated are not an indication for changing or reducing therapy.[8]

While caution is advised in starting beta-blockade (low doses initially so that side-effects can be easily reversed), it is important to titrate dose to effect. In general, the average dose is equivalent to propranolol 80 mg bid, or tds; eg, atenolol 100 mg daily (see Table 6.2). Some, however, will need atenolol 200 mg daily and some will be well on 50 mg daily.

Adverse effects are largely predictable and often caused by inappropriate patient selection. Why prescribe a cardioselective beta-blocker to a patient with bronchospasm when there is a possibility of problems if a nitrate or calcium antagonist can avoid that possibility? Bronchospasm and heart failure are well recognized adverse effects, but cold hands and feet, heavy legs, lethargy and a general washed-out feeling are more frequently experienced. These symptoms reflect a fall in cardiac output (it is not related to cardioselectivity) which is common to all beta-blockers so that they may improve with dosage reduction or transfer to an agent with ISA (eg,

Table 6.2 A practical approach to selecting a beta-blocker for angina*

	Potency	Cardioselective	Optimum dose dynamic half-life hours	Blood–brain barrier penetration	Dosage adjustments
Acebutolol	0.3‡	+†	24	NS	Renal
Atenolol	1	+	24	NS	Renal
Metoprolol	1	+	10–12	Yes	Liver
Nadolol	1.5	0	39	NS	Renal
Oxprenolol	0.5–1‡	0	13	Yes	Liver
Pindolol	6‡	0	8	Yes	None
Propranolol	1	0	8	Yes++	Liver
Sotalol	0.3	0	24	NS	Renal
Timolol	6	0	15	Yes	Liver
Slow oxprenolol	‡		< 24		
Metoprolol SA			24		
Propranolol LA			24		

*How to use this table: Assume propranolol as the reference drug with a potency of 1. Propranolol 80 mg can be given twice daily (half-life 11 hours). It is equal to atenolol 100 mg (potency 1:1) and atenolol can be given once daily (half-life 24 hours). Sotalol is one-third the potency of propranolol so that it needs to be given 240 mg once daily to be equivalent to propranolol 80 mg bid, ie, we compare dosage with 80 mg propranolol equivalent, *not* to total daily dose. †Cardioselectivity of acebutolol is debated. ‡Agents with ISA.

61

acebutolol). Central nervous system side-effects such as muzzy head, loss of memory, poor concentration, vivid dreams (some pleasant, some horrific) and depression also occur and seem to be related to blood-brain passage, which is a greater problem with the lipid soluble (lipophilic) agents. Using a hydrophilic agent (water soluble) these effects may be substantially reduced or even abolished. In turn the lipophilic agents may be better when anxiety is a problem. Noting the mode of excretion of individual beta-blockers, the obvious dose adjustments can be anticipated in patients with significant renal or hepatic disease. Problems can be avoided by using hepatically metabolized drugs in renal failure and renally excreted drugs when there is significant hepatic dysfunction. Similarly, drug interactions may be anticipated if two drugs excreted via hepatic metabolism are used, eg, propranolol and cimetidine. Beta-blockade can lead to impotence in male patients. Although the incidence is less than 10 per cent, and in most studies little more than placebo, routine questioning for side-effects is recommended.

My personal preference is atenolol 50 mg or 100 mg daily given at night if lethargy is a problem. If peripheral side-effects are significant I change to acebutolol 100 mg bid and titrate to effect. If they continue I change to a calcium antagonist. If I am concerned about the possibility of heart failure and nitrates alone are not helpful, I use low doses and the most flexible are propranolol 10 mg tds, or oxprenolol 20 mg tds, titrating carefully. Adding a low dose diuretic (eg, triamterene 50 mg plus hydrochlorothiazide 25 mg once daily) can avoid or control mild failure and allow beta-blockers to continue.

Calcium antagonists

Calcium ions are essential for myocardial contraction and conduction. Calcium antagonists act by impairing the influx of these ions into smooth muscle, myocardial and conducting tissue cells. The four agents available are:

- Verapamil
- Nifedipine
- Diltiazem
- Nicardipine.

	Nicardipine	Nifedipine	Verapamil	Diltiazem
Heart rate	↑	↑	↓↑	↓↑
Atrioventricular conduction	0	0	↓↓	↓
Peripheral vasodilation	+++	+++	++	++
Coronary vasodilation	+++	+++	++	+++
Contractility	↓0	↓0	↓↓	↓

Table 6.3
The calcium antagonists

All act as peripheral vasodilators but important individual differences exist (see Table 6.3). In therapeutic doses, although nifedipine and diltiazem only have a mild effect on cardiac contractility, they must still be used with caution in patients with impaired left ventricular function, especially in the presence of beta-blockade. Claims that nicardipine has no effect on contractility should be viewed with caution.

Many calcium antagonists are under development, eg, nitrendipine and felodipine, and each will need careful assessment.

VERAPAMIL This has a marked action on the atrioventricular node and is consequently a powerful antiarrhythmic drug, particularly for supraventricular tachycardias. In several studies it has been shown to be as effective as beta-blockade in stable angina pectoris.[9] It is not recommended for combined prescribing with beta-blockade because the additive effect on atrioventricular conduction can induce asystole or heart block (see Figure 6.1). It is of great value in patients with obstructive airways disease or peripheral arterial disease where beta-blockade may be contraindicated and where theoretically calcium antagonism may be beneficial. It is effective in doses of 40 mg tds increasing to 120 mg tds. Principal side-effects are flushing and headaches secondary to vasodilation, and constipation (especially in the elderly). Constipation may respond to high fibre diets but can be severe, leading to cessation of therapy. Like beta-blockade verapamil can induce heart failure in those with reduced left ventricular function.

NIFEDIPINE This is a potent arterial vasodilator with no effect on atrioventricular conduction. It is therefore a safe drug to use in combination with beta-blockade, also having

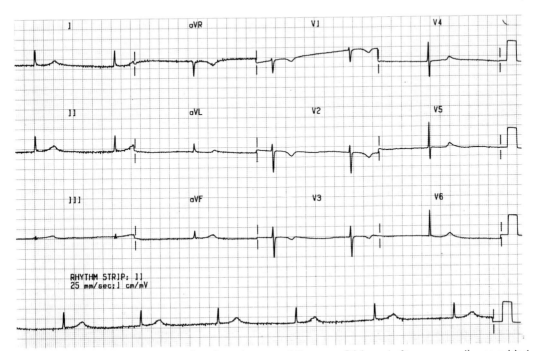

Figure 6.1 Electrocardiogram showing absence of P waves 24 hours after verapamil was added to atenolol. The patient presented asystolic with syncope. She recovered in 48 hours.

less effect in reducing cardiac contraction. Its use as a single agent in angina is surprisingly poorly documented. The possibility of a reflex tachycardia or coronary steal effect renders the need for caution in its use. Several reports detail the need for individual dose titration and the difficulty giving guidelines for drug usage,[10] its failure in the smoking population,[11] and the overall superiority of beta-blockade in comparison.[12] However, the additive effect to beta-blockade is clear and this is where it is believed that its use lies in stable angina. Typical doses are 5 mg tds (in the elderly) increasing to 40 mg bid. Principal side-effects are flushing and peripheral oedema not responsive to diuretics. Headaches may also limit therapy.

DILTIAZEM Available for the past four years, this relatively new agent is similar in profile to verapamil but it has less depressant action on atrioventricular conduction and cardiac contraction. Although it affects atrioventricular conduction, its use in combination with beta-blockade has been reported to be safe.[13] However, caution is still needed when initiating out-of-hospital coprescribing, particularly as the use of nifedipine avoids any risk. Hospital-initiated coprescribing with beta-blockers can be safely continued out of hospital. Diltiazem's clinical effectiveness as monotherapy in stable angina has been established and its reduced side-effect profile (less flushing, less constipation, less peripheral oedema) has been maintained with wide-

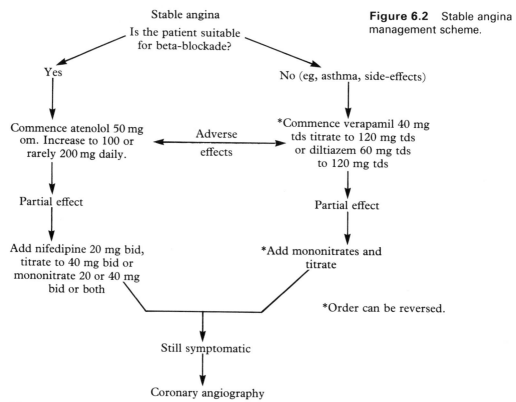

Figure 6.2 Stable angina management scheme.

spread use. The typical starting dose is 60 mg tds increasing to 120 mg tds and it can be used as monotherapy as an alternative to beta-blockade.[14] Like verapamil it is a good alternative to beta-blockade when contraindications or side-effects occur. Because of its efficacy and acceptance by patients, it is assuming the position of calcium antagonist of choice for those with angina pectoris.

NICARDIPINE The latest calcium antagonist is very similar to nifedipine. Most of the literature available is from the pharmaceutical house. While fewer side-effects and lack of depression of left ventricular function are claimed, only small numbers have been evaluated and we must await details of effectiveness in a less selected and therefore more normal population. If the wrong ventricle is selected, no amount of peripheral vasodilatation will offset a depressant effect, but because of the careful selective process for recruitment into hospital trials this is unlikely to be seen. While it is correct to claim an apparent avoidance of depression of cardiac function, this cannot be extrapolated to indicate safety in those with heart failure.

The recommended dose in angina is 20 mg tds titrating to effect with a range of 60–120 mg a day. As with nifedipine some patients will experience pain 30 minutes after therapy and the manufacturers urge caution in those with poor cardiac reserve. There seems to be no advantage over nifedipine and a less convenient dosage regime.

Combination therapy

Although we have only three groups of drugs, no data are available on which is the better in combination. There is no doubt that calcium antagonists and beta-blockers together with nitrates are safe, and triple therapy using nifedipine is safe. However, angina needing this amount of drug control should be investigated further to see if a surgical option is possible (see Figure 6.2). If a surgical option is not possible a scheme might include atenolol 100 mg daily, nifedipine 20 mg bid and isosorbide 5 mononitrate 20 mg bid. The nifedipine and mononitrate can be doubled in most patients and the atenolol occasionally doubled. Combining atenolol with diltiazem in hospital is gaining popularity and the additive beneficial effect is very encouraging. A scheme might include atenolol 100 mg daily, diltiazem 60 mg tds and isosorbide 5 mononitrate 20 mg bid. As for nifedipine, the diltiazem and mononitrate can be doubled.

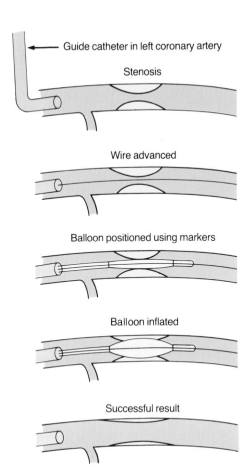

Guide catheter in left coronary artery

Stenosis

Wire advanced

Balloon positioned using markers

Balloon inflated

Successful result

Figure 6.3 The technique of angioplasty.

ANGIOPLASTY

Percutaneous transluminal coronary angioplasty (PTCA) has given the physician for the first time the possibility of increasing the supply of blood to the heart rather than reducing the demand.[15] Unfortunately, in the excitement there has been failure to control the observations and failure to provide satisfactory comparisons with conventional medical therapy or bypass surgery. In 1985 60 000 angioplasties were carried out in the USA but it is not known if optimal therapy was being provided.

The procedure is similar to coronary angiography. The stenosis is identified, a guide wire passed over it and a balloon advanced along the guide wire until it crosses the lesion. The balloon is then inflated and hopefully the stenosis substantially reduced (see Figures 6.3 and 6.4). Currently reported initial success rates are 90 per cent with a recurrence rate at six months of 20–30 per cent. The procedure can then be repeated with a further 80 per cent success rate. As no comparative data exist regarding bypass surgery, historical controls from surgical publications have had to be used. There is no doubt that PTCA is

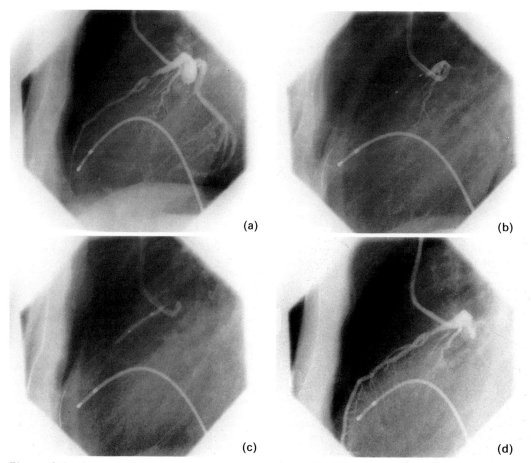

(a) (b) (c) (d)

Figure 6.4 Stenosis before and after angioplasty. (a) Critical stenosis in LAD. (b) Wire across the stenosis to the distal LAD. Balloon across the lesion. (c) Balloon inflated. (d) Successful result.

effective in relieving symptoms and normalizing an abnormal exercise ECG but placing it in a clinical context is difficult.

In single vessel disease there is no difference from surgery initially, but surgery is better at twelve months symptomatically (see Table 6.4). The problem here is that it is known that medical therapy alone is success-

Table 6.4 Comparison of PTCA and surgery in the treatment of single vessel disease

| | Immediate result | | |
	Angioplasty success	Death	Operative infarct
PTCA (per cent)	90 (CABG 6.5)	1	4.9
Surgery (per cent)	—	1	3

| | Follow-up (12 months) | | | |
	Reoperation	Infarct	Death	Asymptomatic
PTCA (per cent)	15 (12 CABG)	2.8	1.4	70
Surgery (per cent)	3	1.5	< 3	90

CABG = coronary artery bypass grafts either immediately because of complications or late because of symptoms. Both PTCA and surgery offer symptomatic benefit compared with conventional medical therapy.

Table 6.5 Comparison of PTCA and surgery in the treatment of multivessel disease

| | Immediate result | | |
	Angioplasty success	Death	Operative infarct
PTCA (per cent)	90 (CABG 4)	1.2	3–5
Surgery (per cent)		2	5

| | Follow-up (12 months) | | | |
	Reoperation	Infarct	Death	Asymptomatic
PTCA (per cent)	27 (15 CABG)	7.3	5.6	64
Surgery (per cent)	3	1.5	3	80

Note the immediate good result but at twelve months the effect is not as sustained as surgery.

ful in single vessel disease and it must be assumed that PTCA is frequently being undertaken on the basis of the 'look' of the lesion rather than the symptoms of the patient or the abnormality of his exercise ECG. In multivessel disease (see Table 6.5) the results are not as impressive when scrutinized carefully, despite the enthusiasm of the PTCA protagonists.[16] One can see a potential major role in the symptomatic, in spite of medical therapy, who are unfit for bypass surgery, which might include patients with severe airways disease or other life-shortening illnesses (eg, cancer). The elderly might be be another group to be considered but here the risks are increased further and caution is advised.[16]

Clearly we are in desperate need of ran-domized controlled trials of PTCA and bypass surgery in varying age groups in patients with stable angina. We have no information on relative risk, longterm efficacy or prognosis versus surgery. Obviously if PTCA is shown to be as good as surgery in various subsets, *and I believe it will be*, it will offer a far less painful therapeutic option for the patient. In the meantime, patients with symptoms and single or multivessel disease involving short (<2 cm) lesions should be considered for PTCA but only if they are provided with an honest appraisal of the plusses and minuses, and the advantages and disadvantages of the surgical option. I currently advocate PTCA on this background with surgical support.

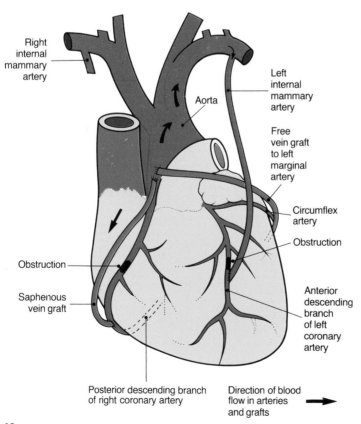

Figure 6.5 A schematic of coronary artery bypass surgery.

Right internal mammary artery

Left internal mammary artery

Aorta

Free vein graft to left marginal artery

Circumflex artery

Obstruction

Obstruction

Anterior descending branch of left coronary artery

Saphenous vein graft

Posterior descending branch of right coronary artery

Direction of blood flow in arteries and grafts

SURGERY

The role of coronary artery bypass surgery in stable angina for relief of symptoms and to lengthen life is well established. It is effective in all age groups and those otherwise fit but over sixty-five years of age benefit as well as the younger patients.[17] In experienced hands the operative mortality is less than 2 per cent. However, with a more complex procedure and an older patient the risk will rise. It is important that patients and relatives fully understand what these figures mean and to put them in a practical realistic context.

The odds are favourable but it should be emphasized that if the patient is one of the 2 per cent the risk to them and their family becomes 100 per cent.

One of the major concerns is the longterm effectiveness of the bypass operation. Attention to risk factors is essential and in the first

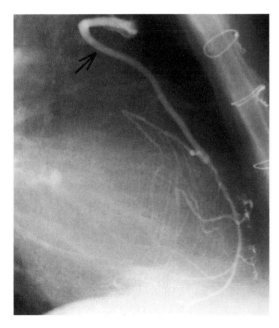

Figure 6.6 Angiogram of successful bypass operation. The vein is arrowed and its point of insertion into the LAD artery clearly leads to good filling of the vessel.

twelve months antiplatelet therapy is also used with either dipyridamole plus aspirin or aspirin alone.[18] This leads to a twelve-month graft patency rate of 85–90 per cent. Atheroma is a relentless disease, however, and surgery bypasses but does not cure the problem (see Figures 6.5 and 6.6).

A ten-year follow-up has shown very encouraging results when the internal mammary artery is used for the bypass procedure with a satisfactory 95 per cent patency rate. This contrasts with only a 50 per cent satisfactory vein condition.[19] Internal mammary grafting is technically more difficult and the artery less suitable in the elderly, so, given the practicalities of life, where possible, the young should undergo artery bypass and the elderly vein bypass.

Morbidity

Patients must be adequately prepared for what lies ahead. Booklets which are designed to explain and prompt questions should be used. All patients should have the operation and aftercare clearly explained to them by the doctors and nurses on the general ward, and be visited pre-operatively by the intensive care staff and physiotherapist. They can expect a 24–48 hour stay in intensive care and an overall nine to ten days' hospital stay. Some will mobilize more quickly than others but a return to work target of three months is set.

Pain from the sternum, leg and back is the major immediate problem. It is treated with generous analgesia but if persistent over several days a non-steroidal anti-inflammatory agent may be needed. The patient can expect intermittent problems for two to three months, mainly chest wall or positional thoracic pain.

Neurological problems of a serious nature (eg, stroke) have been reported to affect 5–6 per cent of patients, with retinal problems in 25 per cent.[20] Major functional disability or death only affected 1–2 per cent of these, however. Psychiatric morbidity is related to pre-operative psychiatric and social maladjustment, neurotic personality traits, and a previous history of psychiatric illness, ie, the operation is not psychiatrically pathological.[21] If the family doctor is aware of problems not readily obvious to the cardiac team, he should alert them in order for a pre-operative psychiatric assessment to be made and careful post-operative care to be provided.

Return to work should be possible at three months. Patients who are most likely to get back to their jobs are under fifty-five years of age. In a depressed economic climate redundancy is all too familiar, so that a failure to get back to work does not correlate with a failed operation.

Some will not want to return to work, and some may have work environment difficulties which preceded the operation and cannot face going back to a conflict causing them lack of enjoyment. Those out of work for longer than six months or those used to heavy work have the greatest difficulty in resuming work. Problems with attitude and confidence can be helped by counselling and a rehabilitation programme is very helpful in this situation (see page 128). Mixing with other people, discussing the problems and visibly getting confidence from supervised exercise represents an option not readily available in the UK but it is an option with very satisfactory results.

No matter what the doctor says, the patient can put it into much simpler words and pass on the information in a much more effective way.

Letter to Viscount Sandon from Sir Edwin Nixon CBE

Dear Dudley

Welcome to the club! As a new member

70

perhaps I could be allowed to mention a few of the rules?

1. Membership is entirely involuntary.
2. There are no meetings.
3. There are no officers or elected officials.
4. Bureaucracy will be kept to a minimum—ideally nil.

There are, however, a number of initiation rites.

a. Stockings will be worn at all times, together with associated suspender devices, for a period of at least six weeks after joining. These must be changed regularly. (Assistance may be sought, and is allowable.)

b. Diet should be controlled and not more than one whisky daily should be consumed.

c. Extraneous wires are inserted into the body, some of which will remain as a permanent reminder of a fractured ribcage.

These initiation rites are supervised by well meaning nurses and doctors.

Although the evidence is not yet conclusive, there is every reason to believe that membership of the club will prolong life beyond average and normal expectations.

Normal life is resumed about three months after induction, usually with a vigour greater than before membership. It is important, however, not to rush into normal life again but to ease one's way into it. (This advice is given to all new members but is rarely taken.)

As a member of the club of eighteen months standing and in spite of the involuntary nature of joining, I can recommend it. I hope in the fullness of time you too will appreciate the benefit.

Look forward to seeing you again.

Yours sincerely

Edwin

PRACTICAL POINTS

- Treating angina is a team approach between patient and doctor.

- Symptoms can be controlled with nitrates, beta-blockers and calcium antagonists.

- Most nitrates are subject to hepatic metabolism but this can be avoided by using a mononitrate preparation.

- Beta-blockade needs to be used to optimal dose and not reduced when asymptomatic resting bradycardia occurs.

- When beta-blockers are contraindicated, use calcium antagonists and/or nitrates.

- Peripheral side-effects of beta-blockers can be reduced by dose reduction or changing to calcium antagonists.

- Diltiazem and verapamil are better as monotherapy, and nifedipine and nicardipine are better in combination with beta-blockade.

- Most adverse effects are caused by inappropriate patient selection; do not take chances.

- Angioplasty is successful in 90 per cent of patients but 20 per cent relapse at six months. Its role versus surgery or medicine is unknown.

- Surgery not only prolongs life for some but relieves symptoms in 80 per cent of those failing to respond to medicine.

- Age should be no barrier to surgery if the patient is otherwise well.

- Surgical mortality averages 2 per cent. For the family, however, a death is 100 per cent.

7
Unstable angina

BACKGROUND

Unstable angina describes a clinical presentation between stable angina and myocardial infarction; it may move in either direction. It has proved difficult to define because it sits between a symptom-related presentation (angina) and a pathological entity (infarction), each of which are dependent on a variety of physiological, psychological and pathological variables.

Many terms continue to be used to cover this syndrome and include the intermediate coronary syndrome, pre-infarction angina, crescendo angina, acute coronary insufficiency and accelerated angina. Clinically the presentation can be divided into three groups:

1   Effort angina of recent onset (less than one month), ie, no previous angina.
2   Changing pattern of angina. Previously stable angina has progressed, increased in frequency and/or severity.
3   Angina at rest for no obvious reason.

While the prognosis is better for groups 1 and 2 (one-third of patients become pain-free) with a reduced risk of infarction and death, angina at rest is associated with higher morbidity and mortality. Patients may unfortunately progress from groups 1 or 2 to group 3.

PATHOPHYSIOLOGY

In the majority of cases severe atheromatous coronary artery disease (CAD) is present. Progression of disease in terms of extent and severity has been documented as the patient moves from a stable to unstable presentation.[2]

The question of coronary artery spasm has arisen initially following the studies of Prinzmetal's variant angina, where ST elevation is a diagnostic feature (see page 77). The role of spasm superimposed on a fixed atheromatous lesion or as an independent factor in the 10 per cent or so who have either minimal or no disease, is debated.[3] There is no doubt it exists; the problem is in defining the extent of its existence (see Chapter 8). In most patients, unstable angina appears to follow fissuring or rupture of an atheromatous plaque with superimposed thrombosis (see Chapter 1). Platelet thrombi may transiently increase the stenosis and cause vasoconstriction. In this way, it represents pathologically a situation between stable angina and infarction.[4] It is impossible without angiography to be certain which mechanism is operating. Fortunately the treatment regimes in the initial phase seem effective across the board of pathologies, so no delay is needed at the start of therapy.

PROGNOSIS

With improved medical therapy there has been a dramatic improvement in prognosis. The mortality in the medically stabilized is 4 per cent at six months with 13 per cent sustaining infarction and 3 per cent cardiac arrest.[5,6] Those presenting with rest pain seem to have a worse prognosis but the data are conflicting. What is certain is that those who fail to respond to treatment have a one month mortality of 20 per cent and up to 40 per cent at one year. A previous history of angina, myocardial infarction and ECG evidence of ischaemia identifies those with a higher morbidity and mortality rate.[7]

The distribution and severity of coronary lesions, as well as the presence of left ventricular dysfunction, also determines prognosis and leads to a recommendation for angiography during the early phase (two weeks) of medical management.[8]

MANAGEMENT

Treatment must be directed at:

- Relief of symptoms
- Prevention of infarction
- Survival.

There is no role for immediate angiography and surgery unless all medical therapy fails. The patient should be started on nitrates, given sublingually out of hospital, and transferred immediately to the cardiac care unit. Here conventional analgesia with intravenous diamorphine is introduced. Because of the debate over the role of spasm, the subsequent management varies from centre to centre. A practical treatment strategy is possible, and can be simple and effective (see Figure 7.1).

Nitrates

These vasodilators reduce oxygen demand as well as benefit coronary spasm (see page 59). Out of hospital they should be given sublingually using isosorbide dinitrate for longer duration of action, to cover the hospital transfer. Buccal nitrates can be added for longer effects. In-hospital intravenous therapy should be started to give rapid blood levels followed by mononitrate 20–40 mg twice daily. Intravenous isosorbide dinitrate 2 mg/hour may be given titrating to effect, providing the systolic blood pressure remains above 90 mmHg. Topical nitrates confer no advantages.

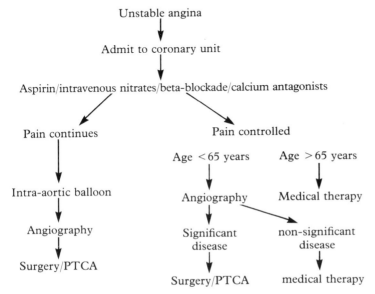

Figure 7.1 Unstable angina management plan.

73

Beta-blockade

The theoretical disadvantage of beta-blockers is that unopposed alpha effects may promote vasoconstriction and they will therefore make the situation worse. The overwhelming evidence, however, supports their effectiveness and in the recent HINT trial they proved superior to nifedipine, which actually led to termination of the trial because the situation worsened.[9]

In those where there are no specific contraindications (bronchospasm, heart failure, resting bradycardia) beta-blockade is routinely initiated. In those already on therapy it is continued or the dose increased. The need for a reduction in the resting heart rate means avoiding agents with ISA (see page 60). Typically atenolol 50 mg should be started (peak blood level 3 hours) increasing to 100 mg or rarely 200 mg daily. Those in pain with a tachycardia and no ST elevation should receive intravenous beta-blockade with atenolol slowly (1 mg/min to 5 mg, or rarely 10 mg).

Beta-blockers may be combined with nitrates, nifedipine, or diltiazem, but not verapamil (see page 63).

Calcium antagonists

Initial enthusiasm for nifedipine as monotherapy has now been tempered.[9,10] Theoretically the reduction in demand and vasodilation should be beneficial but too great an arteriolar dilating effect may lead to the undesirable effect of a coronary steal or reflex tachycardia. While nifedipine can be added effectively to beta-blockade and nitrates it is not advised as the prime agent. Verapamil and diltiazem are effective without too great a vasodilating effect and may slow sinus rate. Verapamil is more likely to depress cardiac contraction (negative inotropy) and atrioventricular conduction. Where beta-blockers are contraindicated these two drugs present a satisfactory option and can be coprescribed with nitrates. Diltiazem may well be safer and

I would use this agent 60 mg tds increasing to 120 mg tds. I am in favour always of avoiding risks.

Aspirin

In doses varying from 300 mg to 1300 mg a day, aspirin reduced the incidence of cardiac death or non-fatal infarction in patients with unstable angina.[11,12] Debate continues over dosage but until there is evidence that lower dosage is effective in practice, 300 mg soluble aspirin daily is recommended for all patients without gastrointestinal contraindications or known hypersensitivity.

Anticoagulation

There are no satisfactory large-scale randomized trials of the effectiveness of anticoagulation. Therapy remains very individual with some administering heparin during the first 48 hours. In the sense that all patients in our cardiac care unit receive 5000 units of heparin subcutaneously 8 hourly to prevent deep venous thrombosis, I admit to using heparin, although I do not advocate the use of higher doses for unstable angina. Given that thrombosis may occur during the unstable episode, thrombolytic agents are currently under study.

Refractory pain

Failure to stabilize the patient with drugs is unusual. Over 80 per cent of patients come under control in the first 48 hours. Continuing pain is a dangerous condition and merits angiography to define suitability for angioplasty or surgery. First, if available, we insert an intra-aortic balloon pump percutaneously (see Figure 7.2). This device requires specialized equipment but by augmenting coronary filling at the same time as reducing demand, pain relief may follow. Angiography is then safer.

Reports of emergency surgery and angioplasty indicate a satisfactory success rate but there is no comparison between the two.[13]

Angioplasty was successful in 93 per cent of cases with no deaths but 7 per cent infarcted. At follow-up restenosis occurred in 28 per cent of patients but good functional capacity was demonstrated in 80 per cent. Coronary surgery is associated with a one month mortality of 1.8–3.5 per cent.[14]

AFTER STABILIZATION Providing medical stabilization occurs, the prognosis in the short term is favourable but, in view of a subsequent infarct rate up to 15 per cent at four months and a 10 per cent mortality at twelve months, I routinely perform angiography about one week after stabilization in patients aged less than sixty-five years. If anatomically at risk by the nature of their coronary lesions and/or degree of left ventricular dysfunction, I advise angioplasty or elective surgery. Follow-up for ten years after surgery is encouraging.[14] Sixty-one per cent are asymptomatic, 20 per cent minimally symptomatic, 14 per cent suffering from angina on ordinary effort and 5 per cent from severe angina. The operative mortality is now 1.8 per cent with a ten-year survival rate of 83 per cent. Reoperation rate is 1.2 per cent per year for the first five years and 2.2 per cent for the next five years. Attention to risk factors post surgery is imperative. These figures should improve with the greater use of the internal mammary artery graft.

Strategy is summarized in Figure 7.1. Management is initially intensive medical therapy. Based on the individual patient and resources of each centre, an investigative approach may or may not be followed. I favour angiography to optimize therapy.

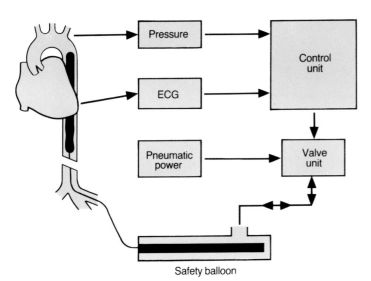

Pressure

ECG

Control unit

Pneumatic power

Valve unit

Safety balloon

Figure 7.2 Intra-aortic balloon pump. The balloon is inserted percutaneously and passed from the femoral artery to the descending aorta. When the heart is in diastole the balloon inflates improving coronary perfusion. When in systole (determined from the ECG) the balloon deflates facilitating cardiac output.

PRACTICAL POINTS

- Unstable angina is effort pain of recent onset, a changing pattern of angina or angina at rest.

- Management strategy is summarized in Figure 7.1.

- Hospital admission is advised.

- Intravenous nitrates form the mainstay of therapy.

- Beta-blockade and calcium antagonists can be added and should be continued if the patient is admitted already taking them.

- Aspirin, if not contraindicated, is begun immediately.

- Angiography is advised to rule out significant disease needing angioplasty or surgery.

8
Variant angina and coronary artery spasm

BACKGROUND

In 1910 Osler[1] suggested that angina was caused by spasm of a large coronary artery but in the ensuing years as the anatomy was defined and obstructive coronary disease recorded this concept fell out of favour. It was Prinzmetal in 1959[2] who, with his description of 'variant' angina, revived the interest. In spite of the explosion of publications since, the role of spasm remains unclear and confused.

DEFINITIONS

Coronary artery spasm is a transient stenosis of a coronary artery leading to myocardial ischaemia in the absence of any obvious increase in myocardial demand, eg, exercise. It is usually immediately reversed by nitrate therapy and may occur in the presence or absence of coronary artery disease (CAD).

Variant angina

This refers to patients who get pain at rest with ST elevation on the ECG. It may occur at the same time every day (at night and early morning being the most common) and be associated with syncope. Exertional angina and CAD may or may not be present. While all patients with variant angina have spasm, spasm itself may be a part of other ischaemic presentations.

INCIDENCE

In variant angina the incidence of spasm is 100 per cent. In patients with unstable angina (associated with ST depression and/or rise)

the incidence is 30–40 per cent.[3] In effort (stable) angina the incidence is 4 per cent.[3]

In patients with acute myocardial infarction it is tempting to allocate the onset of infarction to spasm on a plaque or severe spasm in normal coronary arteries leading to thrombosis. The evidence is speculative and cause and effect have not been established. Comparing nitrates with thrombolysis invariably produces better results with thrombolysis but spasm may then be important in the recanalized vessel (see Chapter 1). At present we have no clear sequence of events that lead to easily defined management plans.

PROGNOSIS (VARIANT ANGINA)

Prinzmetal,[3] following up his original thirty-two patients, recorded a 9 per cent death rate and 38 per cent infarct rate at two years. It is important, however, to make a division between those with normal or near normal coronary arteries, and those with significant obstructive disease. While those who have normal arteries may suffer infarction or death, the incidence is of the order of 8 per cent. By contrast, in those with significant disease the incidence rises to approximately 30 per cent. However, many more of those with coronary disease subsequently develop symptoms and need therapeutic intervention.[4] The impact of new drug techniques with calcium antagonists may influence these figures.

TREATMENT

Coronary vasodilators, principally nitrates and calcium antagonists, are the drugs of first choice in the management of coronary artery spasm. On page 59 the differences between agents and dosage recommendations are made. Again I do not favour nifedipine as monotherapy, preferring diltiazem or verapamil. Combination therapy with calcium antagonists and nitrates may prove effective. In the initial phase intravenous nitrates may be needed.

Beta-blockade remains controversial. Theoretically in the presence of beta-blockade there should be unopposed alpha (vasoconstrictor) activity leading to either the aetiology of spasm or its exacerbation. The overall anti-ischaemic beneficial effects of beta-blockade may counter this, especially in the presence of obstructive coronary lesions and when coprescribed with nitrates or calcium antagonists.

At present a patient with variant angina is admitted to hospital to start intravenous nitrates and oral calcium antagonists. When admitted taking beta-blockers, they are only discontinued if the coronary arteries are known or found to be normal. In other situations a cardioselective agent is preferred (see page 60). Aspirin is introduced (see page 74). Stabilization with oral therapy invariably follows and, when stable, angiography is routinely carried out to assess the anatomy (see Figure 8.1).

Refractory spasm is rare but frightening. It may respond to intra-aortic balloon pumping. If it develops after angiography intracoronary nitrates may be effective (see Figure 8.2).

At present coronary artery surgery appears not to be as successful in comparison with stable angina, with an operative infarct rate

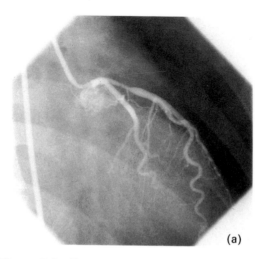
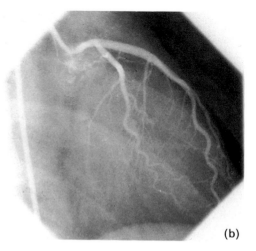

(a)   (b)

Figure 8.1   Coronary artery spasm and its reversal by nitrates. (a) The proximal LAD spontaneously narrowed; (b) improvement in diameter after nitrates.

up to 25 per cent and death rate up to 13 per cent. However, this may improve with perioperative and postoperative calcium antagonists and nitrates which are now routinely used.

Cardiac denervation, either by careful and detailed dissection or removing the heart and returning it (autotransplantation), is a desperate last effort with varying reports of success.[6] Patients needing this are extremely rare. Perioperative and postoperative spasm still occurs and may respond to continuation of medical therapy. I have never seen a case where this highly controversial option has been considered necessary.

PROVOCATION OF SPASM

Ergonovine (ergometrine) has been used to induce spasm and the anatomical response is reproducible in patients with variant angina pectoris.[7] It is dose sensitive and not reproducible in the generalized chest pain population in whom spasm is suspected. While some advocate its regular use and safety, there is a definite morbidity and mortality.[8] Its relevance on a risk:benefit ratio is not obvious and it seems to be a pharmacological rather than physiological exercise. It should therefore not be advocated at all in clinical practice.

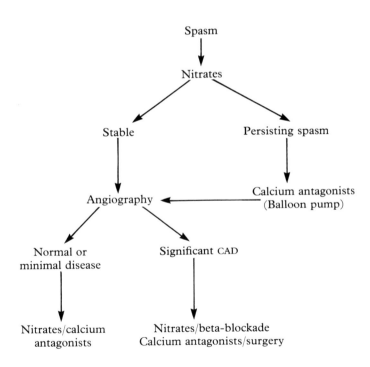

Figure 8.2 Management strategy.

PRACTICAL POINTS

- Coronary artery spasm may occur with and without CAD.

- It is the cause of variant angina.

- It is involved in 30–40 per cent of cases of unstable angina.

- The safest and most rapidly effective drugs are the intravenous nitrates.

- Calcium antagonists are frequently helpful, alone or in combination with nitrates.

- Angiography is advised to rule out significant coronary disease.

- Provoking spasm can be dangerous and is of little clinical relevance.

- If surgery is performed spasm may still recur, so nitrates and calcium antagonists may be used postoperation even if the patient is apparently pain-free.

9
Myocardial infarction—assessment

BACKGROUND

A myocardial infarct represents permanent cellular injury and necrosis after a prolonged ischaemic episode. In the vast majority of cases it follows from a thrombotic occlusion (see page 3) superimposed on atherosclerotic obstructive coronary artery disease (CAD). Rarely infarction follows coronary emboli, spasm, dissection or vasculitis.

HISTORY

The diagnostic features of cardiac pain are discussed on page 31. Acute infarction may develop in a patient with preceding angina. The pain is usually more severe, fails to respond as usual to the use of sublingual nitrates and continues for over 30 minutes. The patient is usually aware of the severity ('the worst pain I've ever had'), often perspires and may vomit or be nauseated. For some the pain comes 'out of the blue' with no obvious warning signs but frequently, on direct questioning, unusual fatigue may have been noticed in the previous few weeks. In diabetics the infarct may be silent, presumably because of a neuropathy. Here unexplained hyperglycaemia (loss of diabetic control) or heart failure should raise the suspicion of infarction. The denervated transplanted heart has a 50 per cent incidence of severe ('accelerated') atheroma after five years and with the wider use of transplantation and better control of rejection, silent infarction may become a frequent problem in this patient group.[1] The presentation is invariably one of heart failure or shock, totally unheralded, in a patient who, until that moment, was apparently progressing well.

The elderly may also suffer acute infarction with few symptoms. Here breathlessness, acute confusion, syncope (a fall, a 'turn') or hemiplegia secondary to embolization may be the only pointers, so a high index of suspicion is essential. A clinical guide is given in Table 9.1.

EXAMINATION

The patient will be in pain which will need immediate therapy with parenteral opiates. Fear and anxiety are always present to a varying degree, not only in the patient but also in those present, whether relatives or friends. Sinus tachycardia may be evident secondary to the pain and fear but as it often reflects heart failure this must also be considered.

The initial presentation may range from almost no haemodynamic problems with a normal examination to severe heart failure (usually acute pulmonary oedema) or cardiogenic shock, (cold, clammy, blood pressure below 80 mmHg systolic, oliguria; see Table 9.2). A slow heart rate is more common with inferior infarcts and may be secondary to increased vagal tone or heart block. Irregular heart beats measured at the apex may suggest extrasystoles or atrial fibrillation. The blood pressure may be raised, normal or low. Hypotension without a rate or rhythm problem is a poor prognostic sign, usually indicating extensive left ventricular damage. The jugular venous pressure may be raised secondary to heart failure, or 'cannon' waves may be visible because of heart block.

Table 9.1 Myocardial infarction — clinical guide

	Symptoms	Comments
Most patients	Retrosternal chest pain 'heaviness', 'tightness', 'weight'. Poor response or failure to respond to nitrates	May radiate to neck, back and arm. Patient may be nauseated and/or perspire
Diabetics	There may be none. Heart failure unexplained	Unexplained diabetic coma should raise suspicion.
Heart transplant	No pain. Failure or shock (sudden death)	Very poor prognosis, urgent retransplant only option
Elderly	May be none. Typical pain and/or breathlessness. Unexplained heart failure	

Table 9.2 Clinical findings

Patient examination	Observation	Comment
1 Normal	Sinus tachycardia >100 beats/min	Pain, fear but think of failure
2 IV sound	S4 S1 S2	Reduced left ventricular compliance
3 III sound Basal crackles	S1 S2 S3	Heart failure
4 Pan systolic murmur (± thrill)	S1 S2 S3	Left sternal edge—VSD
5 Harsh mid to late or pan apical systolic murmur (± thrill)	S1 S2 S3	Acute mitral regurgitation Apex→back
6 Paradoxical second sound (2LIS)	normal: Expiration — S1 A2 P2 / Inspiration — S1 A2 P2; LBBB: Expiration — S1 P2 A2 / Inspiration — S1 P2 A2	
7 Cold, clammy, pale	Systolic blood pressure <80 mmHg Oliguria, 'looks awful'	Cardiogenic shock
8 Hypertension	Fear, pain, known hypertensive	Think of aortic dissection

Palpation may reveal a bulge at the apex caused by systolic paradoxical movement (dyskinesia). Auscultation may be normal or include a IV sound reflecting reduced left ventricular compliance. A III sound and crackles at the lung bases indicates left heart failure. The II sound may be split paradoxically with left ventricular failure or left bundle branch block (LBBB). A harsh pan systolic murmur along the left sternal edge is rare but points to a ruptured ventricular septum (VSD). A harsh mid- to late- or pansystolic apical murmur often radiating to the back suggests either rupture of a mitral cusp or infarction of a papillary muscle. A VSD is more common after anterior infarction and mitral regurgitation after inferior or posterior infarction.

A scratchy rub usually along the sternal edge (see page 38) indicates pericarditis and is present at some time in up to 10 per cent of patients with acute infarcts.

Pulmonary oedema usually indicates more extensive left ventricular damage, though it may follow the mechanical defects of a VSD or acute mitral regurgitation. These may occur without extensive left ventricular damage and therefore with a better prognosis, providing surgical correction is possible.

INVESTIGATIONS

Electrocardiogram

The ECG represents an excellent means of evaluating and recognizing acute myocardial infarction. However, if recorded early enough it may be normal in about one-third of patients.[2] Thus *a normal initial ECG does not rule out infarction or CAD*; however, it does seem to indicate a low likelihood of complications. The comparison of the normal initial ECG with an abnormal initial trace revealed a reduction in life-threatening complications of twenty-three times and death of seventeen times.[2] This may have important practical implications regarding the safety of home care and need for cardiac care unit observation.

The usual sequence of ECG abnormalities (see Figure 9.1) is:

1 ST segment elevation with tall peaked T waves in the leads orientated to the damaged areas—the hyperacute phase of epicardial injury.
2 Q waves appear within hours and ST elevation persists. Pathological Q waves are usually 0.04 seconds or greater in duration and/or to a depth equivalent to 25 per cent of the height of the R wave.
3 In the subsequent days the ST segments gradually return to baseline and T wave inversion occurs.
4 Over weeks the ST segment usually reverts to normal; persistent elevation after six weeks suggests aneurysm formation. Although Q waves usually remain at follow-up, 10 per cent may have normal ECGs.

Problems with ECGs

When previous injury has occurred, new injury adjacent to that site may not be obvious and supportive enzyme data will be required. Similarly problems may occur when a left ventricular aneurysm has led to persistent ST elevation imitating a recent event. Probably the biggest problem is determining the presence of anterior infarction in a patient with LBBB. A Q wave in V1–V3 may be due to either, but a Q in V4 usually points to infarction and a Q wave in V6, I and aVl confirms infarction. Inferior infarcts are not affected by the LBBB.

Infarct localization

Infarcts are categorized into:

- Anterior, which usually involve occlusion of the left coronary artery, in particular the left anterior descending (LAD)
- Inferior, which usually reflect right coronary occlusion but occasionally circumflex occlusion
- Posterior, which may involve the right or circumflex system.

The subdivisions are shown in Table 9.3 in a simplified practical form. Figures 9.2–9.4 show typical twelve-lead ECGs at the time of acute infarction.

Enzymes

In the presence of infarction, enzymes are released into the blood stream. The peak levels indicate the size of the infarct but only

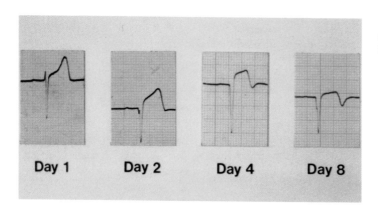

Day 1   Day 2   Day 4   Day 8

Figure 9.1 Evolving changes of myocardial infarction.

Table 9.3 Infarct Localization

Infarct	Leads involved	Possible artery involved
Anterior		
Anteroseptal	V1–V4	LAD
lateral	V5, V6, I, aVl	Diagonal or circumflex
Anterolateral	V1–V6, I, aVl	Proximal LAD/left main
Inferior		
Interior	II, III, aVf	Right coronary artery (RCA)
Inferolateral	II, III, aVf, V5, V6 (I, aVl)	Proximal RCA or circumflex
Inferoseptal	II, III, aVf, V2, V3	RCA or circumflex
Posterior	Tall R waves V1, V2 (V3) (R:S ratio ⩾ 1).	Circumflex or RCA

The anatomical correlation is imprecise but provides a useful guide. Thinking of V1–V4 as anterior, V3 and V4 as septal, V5 and V6, I aVl as lateral and II, III, aVf as inferior enables a logical assessment and description from the resting twelve-lead ECG.

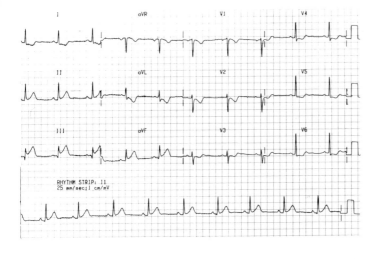

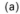

Figure 9.2 Acute inferior infarction. (a) ST elevation in II, III and aVf with reciprocal anterior and lateral ST depression. (b) Within hours a pericardial rub developed and atrial fibrillation which spontaneously reverted to sinus rhythm. (c) Two days later with Q waves and T wave inversion in II, III, aVf. Tall R wave in V2 suggests posterior extension.

(a)

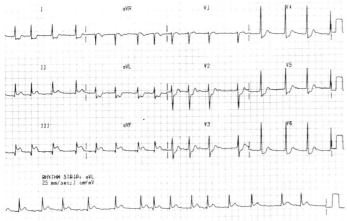

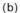

(b)

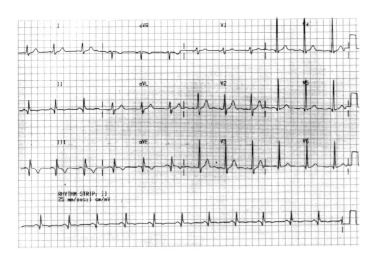

(c)

the cardiac isoenzyme of creatine kinase (CK-MB) is specific for death of myocardium. Enzymes may confirm a clinical suspicion in the absence of ECG changes but usually fulfil a supportive role in establishing the diagnosis.

Total CK (CPK) is present in all skeletal muscle and may rise after intramuscular injections and cardioversion. It can also be raised to twice the normal level in pulmonary oedema without infarction, cerebral trauma and hypothyroidism. CK-MB rises approximately 2 hours after acute infarction, returning to normal after 24–36 hours (see Figure 9.5).

Aspartate transaminase (AST) is also a hepatic enzyme and may be influenced by hepatic congestion due to heart failure. Lactate dehydrogenase (LDH) is of value in checking on a chest pain episode a few days previously.

Because infarction is an acute inflammatory event there may be a neutrophil leucocytosis for 48 hours and the erythrocyte sedimentation rate (ESR) may remain raised for over 10 days.

Chest x-ray

This does not help in the diagnosis but may

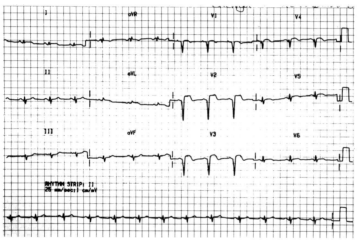

Figure 9.3 (a) Acute anteroseptal infarction. Changes in VI–V4. (b) Routine normal ECG recorded five months previously.

(a)

(b)

identify raised left atrial pressure or frank pulmonary oedema. In the presence of anterior infarction, high CK levels and arrhythmias, radiological and clinical evidence of failure is more likely.[3] A wide mediastinum may suggest dissection, especially if fluid is seen at the lung base.

OTHER POSSIBLE TESTS

Myocardial imaging (see page 52)
This can be helpful when diagnosis is in doubt, but usually requires transport of the patient to special facilities.

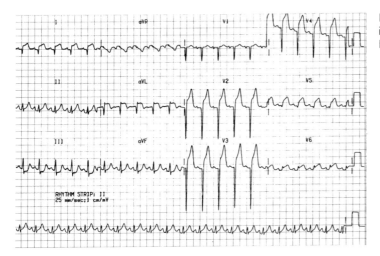

Figure 9.4 Anterolateral infarction. Changes in V2–V6, I and aVI.

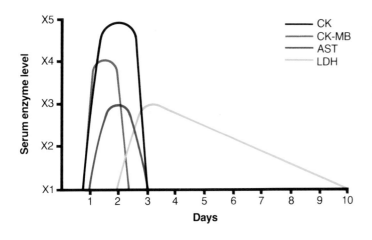

Figure 9.5 Serum enzyme elevation in acute myocardial infarction. AST=Aspartate transaminase; CK=creatine kinase; CK-MB=isoenzyme for cardiac muscle; LDH=lactate dehydrogenase.

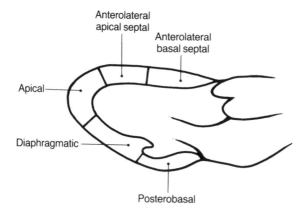

Anterolateral
apical septal

Anterolateral
basal septal

Apical

Diaphragmatic

Posterobasal

Figure 9.6 Schematic representation of echocardiographic images of left ventricular wall movement.

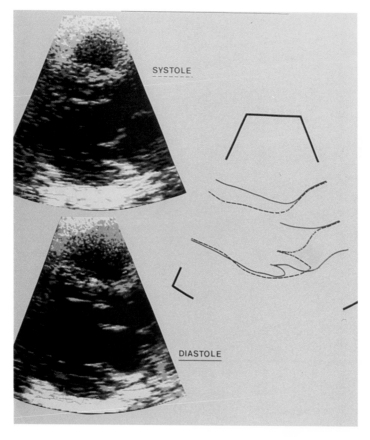

SYSTOLE

DIASTOLE

Figure 9.7 Echocardiogram after acute inferior myocardial infarction. The posterobasal and diaphragmatic segments are akinetic.

'Hot spot'

Intravenous technetium (^{99m}Tc) pyrophosphate precipitates as calcium complexes in the four days after acute infarction.[4] Its sensitivity is 90 per cent for the detection of acute infarction.

'Cold spot'

Areas of severely decreased myocardial perfusion at rest are shown by thallium-201 with a sensitivity of 90 per cent when administered in the first 24 hours.[5]

Echocardiography

This has been used to detect left ventricular segmental dysfunction and changes may precede ECG or CK appearances.[6] The machine can be brought to the bedside or used in the emergency room. Two-dimensional echocardiography provides a complete and spatially oriented view of left ventricular function (see Figure 9.6). Wall movement abnormalities can be seen easily (see Figure 9.7) and, given that they occasionally precede ECG or enzyme changes, the potential for early intervention with a view to infarct size limitation using echocardiography needs exploration. It remains true to say that the principal role of echocardiography is in evaluating the complications of myocardial infarction, which will be discussed later.

PRACTICAL POINTS

- Myocardial infarction is principally diagnosed on history.

- It is confirmed by ECG and enzyme rises.

10
Myocardial infarction—pre-hospital management

BACKGROUND

As there are 500 000 acute infarcts in the UK annually and as the vast majority occur out of hospital, the pre-hospital phase of management is crucial. Given that between 30 and 40 per cent will die, many from reversible ventricular fibrillation within the first 2 hours, the opportunity for a substantial impact on reducing sudden deaths rests in the community.

Ideally a fully trained team should be in the home within the first hour, and preferably the first few minutes, and they should carry full resuscitation equipment. This means that the community must be able to recognize the chest pain for what it is and respond quickly. It is estimated that if immediate coronary care was applied to urban areas only and the population was educated in resuscitation about 5000 lives could be saved annually.

> While my daughter was queuing at the checkout of a supermarket a man in front of her apparently had a heart attack. She gave him mouth-to-mouth resuscitation and heart massage but the man died.
>
> In a crowded shop my daughter was the only one who gave assistance. Nobody helped to keep people away. The checkout clerk continued to check people through and people walked over my daughter while she was attempting to revive the man.
>
> What a world we live in if out of a shop containing 1000 people only one person was brave or sensible or caring enough to give some assistance to a dying man. (Letter to *The London Evening Standard*, April 29 1986)

In Auckland, New Zealand, coronary ambulances take a mean time of 6 minutes to reach the patient and thirty to forty patients a year are resuscitated outside hospital and survive to go home.[1] The response time and service in the UK is patchy.[2] The best is represented by Brighton where the coronary ambulance response time averages 5 minutes, and 25–30 patients are resuscitated and survive to leave hospital and return home each year.

Out-of-hospital care was pioneered in Seattle using the fire brigade and paramedics. In the USA paramedics undergo full training and are a recognized and respected profession. In the UK the government has not encouraged these services, paramedics are not trained fully and their job is not prestigious or well paid. There is no doubt that a standardized degree course is needed in the UK so that when qualified, the paramedics will be recognized by authority (medical and nonmedical) as the essential first-line to an incident needing or potentially needing resuscitation skills. Where centres exist, resuscitation rates of 20–100 per year are recorded for a population of about 350 000[2] (see Figure 10.1). It is hoped that DHSS-recognized training schemes will begin operating in 1987.

The community must be educated to act before specialists arrive, practitioners may be in the front line, especially in rural practices, and must know what to do. The arrival of a resuscitation ambulance completes the team for taking coronary care of the most vulnerable pre-hospital phase of acute myocardial infarction.

The following guidelines should help the family doctor called to the chest-pain patient.

IMMEDIATE CARE

A practitioner who wishes to take on the responsibility of acute coronary management outside hospital should have access to an ECG machine and a defibrillator and he must be familiar with the basics of resuscitation. In other situations he must respond with the fundamentals of acute coronary care.

RELIEF OF PAIN

The patient may have already taken his nitrates, which may have had no effect or modified the pain. If not, nitrates should be tried and the nitrate spray preparation, which is rapid acting and has a shelf-life of three years, lends itself to transport in the doctor's bag. There is no doubt, however, that opiates should be administered intravenously as soon as possible. The rapid pain relief which follows has a major psychological as well as physical benefit, with a further beneficial effect on venous return to the heart. Diamorphine and morphine are preferred, pethidine has unpredictable haemodynamic effects and pentazocine adverse haemodynamic effects which may lead to pulmonary oedema. Morphine 10 mg and cyclizine 50 mg/ml is available as a convenient general practice ampoule, with the necessary antiemetic to counteract the adverse effect of the opiates. If chosen, a half ampule (0.5 ml, 5 mg morphine, 25 mg cyclizine) should be injected followed by the

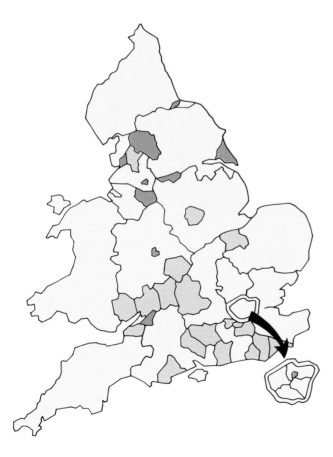

Figure 10.1 Resuscitation ambulances in the UK. Brown areas indicate where ambulances are crewed only by ambulance men and light brown areas doctors or nurses. Courtesy of Richard Vincent.

remainder if pain persists at 10 minutes. Otherwise, diamorphine 5 mg by slow intravenous injection is recommended, followed by a further 2.5 mg at 10 minutes if severe pain persists. Reduce the dose by half if airways disease has been a chronic problem. Cyclizine 50 mg is preferable as the antiemetic because of its central mode of action. There is no evidence that diamorphine is superior to morphine—the policy is one of standardization.

Some centres have used inhaled nitrous oxide to relieve ischaemic pain.

HOME OR HOSPITAL

Once the pain has been relieved, the decision remains whether to transfer to hospital or manage at home. In Table 10.1, the options and reasons are summarized. The principal risk is ventricular fibrillation in the first few hours. The risk is maximal in the first 1–2

Table 10.1 Myocardial infarction — home or hospital?

Hospital	Reason
Within 6 hours definitely and 12 hours probably	Ventricular fibrillation therapy
Age less than 65 years	Active member of community
Complications	Heart failure, shock, heart block
Housing	Lives alone, spouse needs to work, not restful
Other medical problems	Diabetes, stroke

Home	Reason
Elderly patient	Do not respond well to environment change
Over 6 hours and well	Problems unlikely
Other illness	Cancer etc.

hours, receding after 6 hours. If the doctor has any doubt the patient should be transferred. If the doctor cannot guarantee regular visits or if social circumstances are unsuitable, the patient should be transferred, and if the patient and family feel 'safer' in hospital that feeling should be respected. Cardiac care units have reduced the mortality from 25 per cent to 10–15 per cent. They pool trained staff, optimize management, identify risks and capitalize on therapeutic advances. However, some patients will do as well at home. The elderly do not respond as well to hospital transfer and those who have other life-limiting disease (eg, cancer) are unlikely to wish to leave their homes. An infarct *without* problems that occurred over 12 hours before the visit can be safely managed at home if the patient and doctor are happy with the arrangement.

BLOOD PRESSURE

A raised blood pressure may reflect pain or anxiety and usually responds to analgesia. Persistent hypertension indicates the need for hospital transfer for management and exclusion of a dissecting aneurysm. Hypotension of less than 100 mmHg systolic may reflect shock (clammy, pallid) or an arrhythmia and requires hospital transfer for specific therapy.

HEART FAILURE

This is an adverse prognostic sign. If pulmonary congestion occurs the mortality is increased five times, if systemic hypoperfusion occurs (shock) it is increased eleven times and if both occur it is increased twenty-five times.[3] For signs of congestion, frusemide 40 mg iv should be administered and the patient transferred. If the blood pressure is adequate, nitrates may also be given, eg, isosorbide 5 mononitrates 20 mg orally. If the patient is an elderly man check for prostatic symptoms and give frusemide 20 mg iv to try to avoid the risk of acute retention of urine.

ARRHYTHMIAS

Undue bradycardia (less than fifty beats/minute) or a rate of less than sixty/minute with a poor haemodynamic state is a cause for concern. The slow rhythm may lead to ventricular fibrillation. The legs should be raised and atropine injected in 300 μg doses to effect or 1.2 mg. The low dose approach is essential because a small amount of vagal activity (bradycardia) can mask a major amount of sympathetic activity (tachycardia). Giving too much atropine may lead to a much worse situation with a tachycardia and ventricular irritability.

Sinus tachycardia (rate > 100 beats/minute) results from sympathetic overactivity. However, it is also a warning sign of heart failure. If associated with ventricular extrasystoles, lignocaine 100 mg iv or 300 mg im should be given before transfer. Preloaded syringes are available. Doubts still remain concerning the safety of routine pre-hospital lignocaine but in a recent study of 400 mg im lignocaine into the deltoid muscle the incidence of ventricular fibrillation was significantly reduced at 15 minutes when adequate plasma concentrations were achieved, as was ventricular tachycardia.[4] Furthermore, adverse effects were slight though non-fatal asystole did occur. However, only 30 per cent of the patients enrolled in the study had sustained an infarct and mortality was not affected because the ambulances carried defibrillators. It has been calculated that 150 patients will need therapy to protect one from ventricular fibrillations.[5]

Current recommendation for heart rates above 80–100 beats/minute would be that lignocaine is indicated if there are extrasystoles, and if there is no haemodynamic depression which lignocaine could make worse. The drug should be given 100 mg iv or 250–400 mg im depending on body size. If in doubt do not give it. Because it is metabolized by the liver, reduce the dose by half if there is a history of chronic liver disease.

If there is no ECG available, identifying rhythm problems is difficult. Ventricular tachycardia is faster than 130 beats/minute but so is supraventricular tachycardia. Carotid sinus massage (only safe when a defibrillator is present) (see Figure 10.2) does not slow ventricular tachycardia so lignocaine should be used. If there is a slow pulse it should be checked at the apex to clarify whether it is a genuine bradycardia or pulse deficit due to a more irregular rhythm. All patients with arrhythmias should be transferred to hospital.

In Table 10.2 a useful cardiac drug pack for out-of-hospital use is summarized.

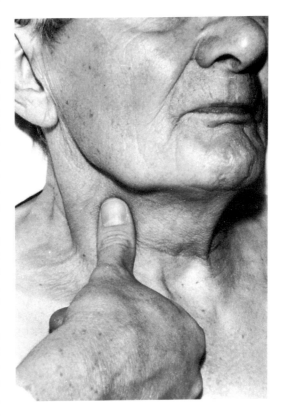

Figure 10.2 Carotid sinus massage. The sinus is massaged (not in patients with carotid bruits) in the presence of a defibrillator for 5 seconds with firm pressure but insufficient to occlude the ipsilateral temporal artery pulse.

Table 10.2 Cardiac drug pack for general practice

Drug (generic name)	Dose	Use
Morphine 10 mg + cyclizine 50 mg/ml	0.5–1 ml iv	Pain relief
Atropine	300–2400 µg iv	Undue bradycardia
Lignocaine	100 mg iv	Ventricular arrhythmias
	300 mg im	+ prophylaxis for ventricular fibrillation
Nitrate spray	2 sprays to buccal mucosa	Pain relief
Sodium bicarbonate 8.4 per cent	50 ml	During resuscitation
Adrenaline	10–50 ml 1:10 000 iv	Asystole
Frusemide	20–80 mg iv	Pulmonary oedema
Salbutamol inhaler	Up to 4 inhalations	Bronchospasm
Aminophylline	250 mg slowly iv	Pulmonary oedema Bronchospasm

PRACTICAL POINTS

- Pain relief should be as quick as possible. Use nitrates and intravenous opiates with cyclizine.

- Hospital care is preferred for most patients.

- A simple drug pack will suffice for most events.

- The basics of first aid and resuscitation may save many lives.

11
Myocardial infarction—resuscitation

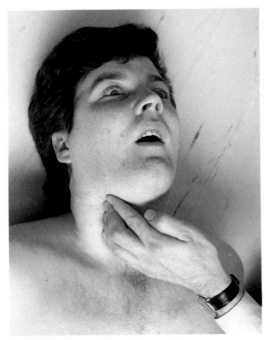

Figure 11.1   Feeling the carotid pulse.

BACKGROUND

The need to be able to manage and cope with a resuscitation exists both inside and outside hospital. It invariably affects the first 6 hours postinfarction when it is a primary event. Sudden death may occur without infarction but the resuscitation procedures are the same.

ASSESSMENT

The typical situation is that of a collapsed patient. The old mnemonic is still valid:

- A = Airway
- B = Breathing
- C = Chest compression
- D = Definitive therapy.

First be sure this is an arrest and not just a faint. Shout at the patient 'Are you OK?' Check if he is breathing and the carotid pulse to see if there is an output (see Figure 11.1).

Figure 11.2   Recovery position.

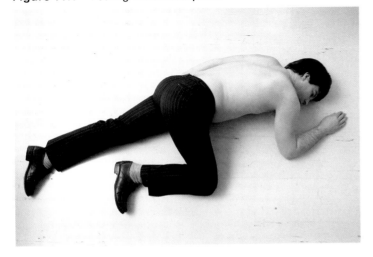

The carotid is better than the femoral as a judge of output since it is rarely absent secondary to arterial disease. The carotid is identified by pressing backwards onto the cervical spine, next to the laryngeal cartilage.

CAFE CORONARIES

Check for airways obstruction caused by a fishbone, for example. The patient makes a choking, gasping noise and may stop breathing before the pulse stops. If the patient is still conscious, encourage him to cough vigorously. Get him to lean on a chair and thump him on the back. Alternatively approach the patient from behind and provide firm abdominal pressure (the Heimlich manoeuvre). If unconscious, extend the neck with the patient supine on the floor. If there is still no airway, open the mouth and search with the fingers for any obstruction. Remove dentures and insert an airway if available. When breathing, place the patient in the recovery position (see Figure 11.2) which causes the tongue to fall forwards and vomit to run out of the mouth.

CARDIOPULMONARY ARREST

Act quickly—place the patient supine on a hard surface. Call out for help; instruct others to dial the emergency code, 999 for the UK, or the hospital team, whichever is appropriate.

1   **THE PRAECORDIAL BLOW (see Figure 11.3)**   Strike the patient forcefully two or three times before moving him into the resuscitation position. There is an outside chance of interrupting ventricular fibrillation and restarting asystole.[1] It is relatively quick and harmless.

2   **CLEAR THE AIRWAY, REMOVE DENTURES**   Begin mouth-to-mouth ventilation (see Figure 11.4). The neck should be extended to open the airway, the mouth-to-mouth seal should be tight and the nose

clamped. If suction is available use it to clear out any blood or vomit. Remember after breathing in to allow for air exit by removing your mouth or unclamping the nose. Insert an airway if available (see Figure 11.5) and intubate if in hospital.

3   **CHEST COMPRESSION (IE, CARDIAC MASSAGE) SHOULD BEGIN IMMEDIATELY**   If the thump and four quick breaths have produced no pulse the chest must be compressed (see Figure 11.6). The lower sternum is compressed with the heel of the hands with the arms straight. Aim for sixty compressions a minute if single handed. If two people are involved shout out your drill (every resuscitator is different); 'I'm going fifteen to two' means fifteen compressions to two inhalations. Check the effectiveness of massage by palpation of the peripheral pulses.

DEFIBRILLATION

This is routine hospital treatment and most defibrillators now have the ability to record the ECG via the paddles, avoiding losing time while applying leads. Out of hospital the defibrillator may not arrive so basic resuscitation first aid must be used to maintain the circulation during the transfer to hospital. This can be exhausting and the load must be shared. If resuscitation begins early enough there remains a chance of success and it must be carried on even though it seems a long time—do not procrastinate.

Ventricular fibrillation

This is the commonest and most correctable cause of cardiac arrest secondary to acute myocardial infarction. I would recommend you use the defibrillator as soon as it arrives—quickly and blind of the rhythm; if it is ventricular fibrillation it may reverse it, if it is asystole it will do no harm or good. I give one shock of 200 joules. If there is no pulse after 3 seconds, compression is continued while the ECG is recorded. The procedure then depends on the rhythm. While all this is going on compression and ventilation must continue. All too often the team stands back while the ECG trace is established.

Technique

POSITION   One electrode is placed below the right clavicle and the other at the apex (see Figure 11.7). Electrode jelly or pads reduce the impedance at the interface between plate and skin and prevent burning. If jelly is used it must be localized and not form a bridge between the paddles. KY jelly has a high resistance to current flow and is not suitable.

PROCEDURE   The person holding the paddles is responsible not just for the patient but the lives of the team helping. He must *shout* 'All off' or 'Everyone clear'. He must check the anaesthetist is away. Blood, urine, saline, rainwater and metal act as conductors. Check that you as the operator are clear as well as everyone else.

SALUTARY TALES

1   An arrest occurred in hospital. The registrar shouted 'All clear'. He delivered the shock and his senior house officer (SHO) fell over in ventricular tachycardia. The patient's foot was in contact with the metal arrest trolley upon which the SHO was leaning. The registrar successfully defibrillated his SHO and the patient recovered also.

2   An arrest occurred in the hospital car park. The patient was half in and half out of the car. It was raining. All the members of the team were touching the car. Fortunately I was walking past, saw the situation and shouted 'stop!'. A consultant cannot afford to lose his entire team as a result of one shock!

DEFINITIVE THERAPY

Ventricular fibrillation   (see Figure 11.8)

This is the most common cause of cardiac arrest in the ischaemic patient.[2] It may occur within the first few hours after myocardial infarction (primary ventricular fibrillation) and be associated with either little or substantial myocardial damage. Late onset fibrillation (secondary) usually relates to cardiogenic shock or severe heart failure (ie, extensive muscle loss) and has a poor prognosis. The primary electrical event can be reversed in 80 per cent, the secondary in only 20 per cent.

While very rarely sinus rhythm is restored spontaneously, drugs alone have no proven effect in abolishing the ventricular fibrillation once established. A dc shock is the definitive therapy.

Technique for a typical arrest

1   Arrest detected—First-aid, call for help, establish iv line.
2   Defibrillation 1×200 joules blind, compression continues afterwards for 10 seconds
3   Check output—If none spontaneously, apply chest compression for at least fifteen compressions
4   Read ECG—Ventricular fibrillation
5   Repeat shock at 200 joules and if no success at 400 joules following above sequence
6   Read   ECG—Ventricular fibrillation. Lignocaine 100 mg iv. Sodium bicarbonate 8.4 per cent 50 ml after 15 minutes of arrest
7   Defibrillate 400 joules—Follow above sequence
8   Read   ECG—Ventricular fibrillation. Continue massage and ventilation. Check potassium, check acidosis and correct

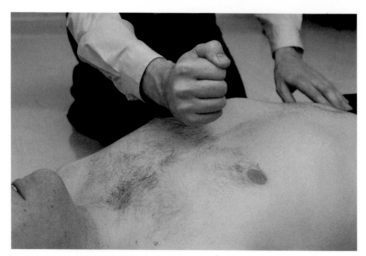

Figure 11.3   The praecordial blow.

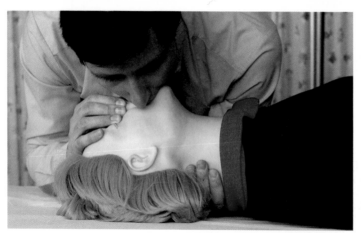

Figure 11.4   Artificial (mouth-to-mouth) ventilation.

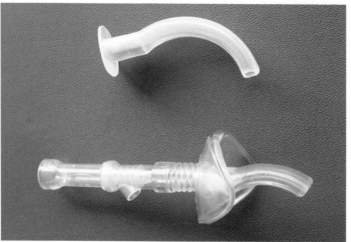

Figure 11.5   The two most commonly used airways: Guedel (above) and Brook (below). New airways are being developed.

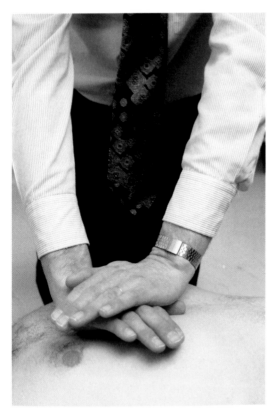

Figure 11.6 External cardiac massage.
Pressure is delivered to the lower sternum.

9 Is ventricular fibrillation fine?—Give adrenaline 10 cc of 1 in 10 000 strength and shock

10 Is ventricular fibrillation coarse (high amplitude)?—Give 100 mg iv lignocaine + shock and/or give procainamide 50–100 mg iv and/or bretylium 500 mg iv and/or amiodarone 300 mg iv and shock after each

11 At this point the situation is desperate and a successful result unlikely. Consider ceasing efforts now if no success.

Points

1 After a dc shock there is always a period of asystole. Do not correct this until 1 minute after the shock for fear of reverting to ventricular fibrillation.

2 Administer drugs as centrally as possible. Peripheral venous stasis may lead to peripheral pooling of drugs. The endotracheal route is effective for lignocaine and adrenaline but not bicarbonate (twice intravenous doses are needed).

3 Recurrent ventricular fibrillation may follow insertion of a pacemaker wire. Try to reposition or if necessary remove it.

Figure 11.7 The usual electrode position for defibrillation.

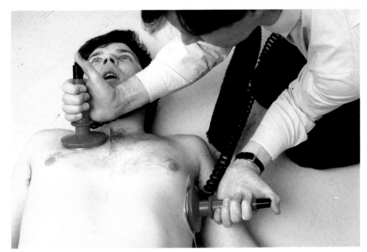

SUCCESS

If sinus rhythm is established lignocaine should be infused for 24–48 hours. After the boluses already given, administer 4 mg/hour for 1 hour then 2 mg/minute. Consider dexamethasone 10 mg iv to reduce cerebral oedema. If lignocaine is ineffective try procainamide, 100 mg iv per minute up to 1 g, then 2 mg/minute by infusion.

If the patient is in sinus rhythm but has a poor output he has a poor prognosis. Cautious dopamine and/or dobutamine infusion may improve the circulation but carries the risk of inducing further ventricular fibrillation. It may be necessary to stabilize the situation with ventilation and/or intra-aortic balloon pump.

For most patients ventricular fibrillation is a potentially fatal rhythm disturbance which responds to defibrillation satisfactorily but, unfortunately, substantial numbers of possible survivors die as a result of lack of equipment and trained individuals.

ASYSTOLE

About 25 per cent of hospital and 10 per cent of out-of-hospital arrests are asystolic.[3] The prognosis is poor.

Asystole implies loss of all ventricular activity (see Figure 11.9). It is imperative to check the ECG connections, the gain switch on the monitor and the switch position. If monitoring via the paddles, the switch is of no use if pointing to a lead selection.

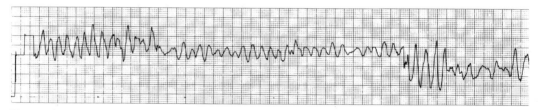

Figure 11.8 Ventricular fibrillation.

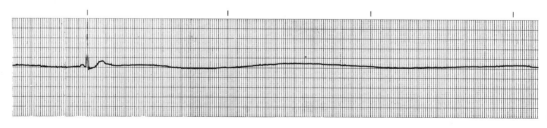

Figure 11.9 Asystole. (The marks at the top of the trace indicate three-second intervals.)

MANAGEMENT

It is always worth trying atropine to reverse any excess of vagal (cholinergic) activity. I use 1.2 mg iv. Of course compression and respiration are essential. Specific drug therapy involves the immediate use of adrenaline 10 cc of 1 in 10 000 which may be repeated. Calcium choloride is always given though doubts have been expressed concerning its efficacy and it is now not recommended by the British Cardiac Society or the American Heart Association for asystole.

The role of pacing is debated but is recommended in the younger age group or when transient returns of rhythm are noted. The new transthoracic noninvasive systems (though uncomfortable) may buy time for a definitive venous system to stabilize the situation. The advantage is that they can be applied anywhere without x-ray screening (see Figure 11.10) and used during hospital transfer.

If a satisfactory rhythm is restored it may be necessary to provide inotropic support afterwards (see page 107).

Electromechanical dissociation

This means there is a co-ordinated ECG rhythm but no output. It is imperative to exclude mechanical factors. The most correctable is tamponade caused by blood in the pericardium. Also consider a massive pulmonary embolus, tension pneumothorax or severe blood loss from elsewhere, eg, ruptured abdominal aneurysm.

Treatment is to follow the pattern for asystole but here calcium may be of more use. I *always* advance a needle to the pericardium to make sure there is no tamponade before I abandon resuscitation.

Discontinuing efforts

One person has to be in charge and responsible: this is the most senior medical doctor present, in hospital usually the registrar. Out of hospital this decision is very difficult if no apparatus is available. If first aid has been initiated within the first 4 minutes (ie, the brain may be alive) efforts should continue until hospital transfer.

The decision to abandon efforts must be positive:

1 Have all efforts been tried including drug options for ventricular fibrillation?
2 Have mechanical causes been excluded?
3 Was hypothermia a component initially, eg, drowning? If so try for longer.
4 Is the ventricular fibrillation recurrent with good output between? In hospital insert a balloon pump. Think of overdrive pacing (ie, pacing over 140 beats/minute).
5 Do you get an ECG but no output every time? Hopeless usually.
6 Are the pupils fixed and dilated? This indicates cerebral circulation is ineffective.
7 Does any member of the team feel unhappy to stop—if so why?
8 Discontinue with a positive statement: 'OK. We have tried everything, there is no output. Let us retire gracefully'.
9 Remember death is not a failure but a part of life; it is necessary to be kind in death as well as in life.
10 Talk to the relatives, thank the helpers, particularly praise any young nurses who may be upset or new to an arrest.
11 Accurately record the events in the notes in red ink; inform the coroner if necessary.

SUMMARY

Figure 11.11 summarizes a practical approach to a cardiac arrest. If resuscitation is successful after ventricular fibrillation, the patient is often well quickly but needs pain relief and stabilization. Some cases may be more complicated, with a low blood pressure needing more detailed assessment. All cases should enter a cardiac care unit for monitoring. If complicated, blood gases and potassium levels should be measured and corrected if abnormal. If the blood pressure is low a urinary catheter should be inserted for fluid balance and to check the response to inotropic agents. If there is a haemodynamic problem a central venous pressure or a Swan-Ganz pulmonary artery catheter should be inserted to monitor fluid volume. If the patient has signs of cerebral damage he may need diazepam for convulsions or dexamethasone to reduce oedema.

All patients undergoing chest compression should have a chest x-ray examination to exclude a traumatic pneumothorax.

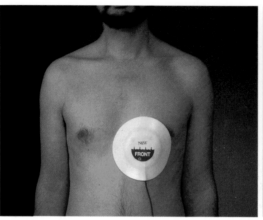 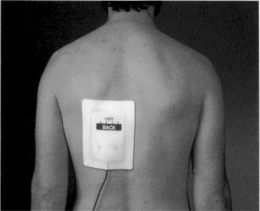

Figure 11.10 Transthoracic pacing. One electrode is placed on the front of the chest and one on the back.

CARDIOPULMONARY RESUSCITATION

DRUGS

All doses based on 70 kg. man.

	Intravenous	Endotracheal	Comment
ADRENALINE	10 ml of 1:10,000	20 ml of 1:10,000	
ATROPINE	1 mg	2 mg	
BRETYLIUM TOSYLATE	500 mg	—	Slow injection
CALCIUM CHLORIDE	10 ml of 10%	—	Must not be injected with bicarbonate
ISOPRENALINE	100 µg	—	Infusion 2 mg in 500 ml 5% Dextrose Rate as appropriate
LIGNOCAINE	100 mg	200 mg	3 mg/min I.V.
SODIUM BICARBONATE	50 ml of 8.4%		Not as Routine. Only refractory cases pH to be measured as soon as possible

THE RESUSCITATION COUNCIL (UK)

Published and printed by Asmund S. Laerdal, Stavanger, Norway 1984
Available from Laerdal Medical Ltd. Orpington Kent U.K.

© The Resuscitation Council UK 1984

00332 EN

Figure 11.11 Cardiopulmonary resuscitation. Two self-adhesive posters provided by the Resuscitation Council. (Free copies obtainable from Laerdal Medical Ltd, Orpington, Kent, UK).

CARDIOPULMONARY RESUSCITATION

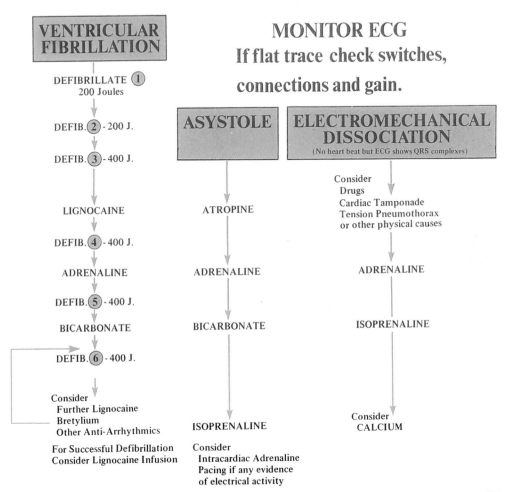

VENTRICULAR FIBRILLATION

DEFIBRILLATE ① 200 Joules

DEFIB. ② - 200 J.

DEFIB. ③ - 400 J.

LIGNOCAINE

DEFIB. ④ - 400 J.

ADRENALINE

DEFIB. ⑤ - 400 J.

BICARBONATE

DEFIB. ⑥ - 400 J.

Consider
Further Lignocaine
Bretylium
Other Anti-Arrhythmics

For Successful Defibrillation
Consider Lignocaine Infusion

MONITOR ECG
If flat trace check switches,
connections and gain.

ASYSTOLE

ATROPINE

ADRENALINE

BICARBONATE

ISOPRENALINE

Consider
Intracardiac Adrenaline
Pacing if any evidence
of electrical activity

ELECTROMECHANICAL DISSOCIATION
(No heart beat but ECG shows QRS complexes)

Consider
Drugs
Cardiac Tamponade
Tension Pneumothorax
or other physical causes

ADRENALINE

ISOPRENALINE

Consider
CALCIUM

THE RESUSCITATION COUNCIL (UK)

Published and printed by Asmund S. Laerdal, Stavanger, Norway 1984 ·
Available from Laerdal Medical Ltd. Orpington Kent U.K.

© The Resuscitation Council UK 1984

00333 EN

PRACTICAL POINTS

- This chapter is practical throughout. Resuscitation should be understood fully.

12
Myocardial infarction—hospital care

BACKGROUND

Hospital care can be divided into general measures forming the routine policy of the unit and specific treatments needed for complications. This latter area is changing rapidly with the use of thrombolysis. The King's College Hospital Cardiac Care Guide is reproduced in note form in Appendix 1.

General therapy: cardiac care unit

The psychological aspects are discussed on page 128.

ANALGESIA

This may have been administered out of hospital (see page 91). The relief of pain provides psychological relief as well as physical comfort. It reduces output from the sympathetic nervous system which may be having adverse effects on myocardial oxygen demand by increasing heart rate, blood pressure and cardiac contractility.[1]

All patients receive intravenous opiates. I give diamorphine 5 mg by slow intravenous injection. Increments of 2.5 mg iv after 10 minutes may be necessary. The patient with chronic respiratory disease should have dosages halved to try to avoid excessive depression of the respiratory centre. To avoid nausea or vomiting, cyclizine 50 mg iv is given per 5 mg of diamorphine. There is no place for intramuscular injections in hospital; they are needlessly painful, slower acting and interfere with total creatine phosphokinase (CPK) estimations by raising levels from skeletal muscle.

Patients are prescribed diamorphine 5 mg iv with cyclizine 4 hourly as necessary. For persistent pain it is first necessary to exclude pericardial pain. This is typically worse on deep inspiration and a rub may be audible (see page 38). It responds rapidly to soluble aspirin 600 mg 6 hourly or indomethacin 25–50 mg tds. If the patient has a past history of peptic ulcer an H_2 antagonist (ranitidine 150 mg bid or cimetidine 400 mg tds) should be used in addition.

If the pain is ischaemic, intravenous nitrates should be used after an initial trial of sublingual therapy. Glyceryl trinitrate (5–200 µg/minute) or isosorbide dinitrate (2 mg/hour titrating) are instituted and increased to pain relief effect or a fall in systolic blood pressure below 90 mmHg. Patients with pain without heart failure, especially if there is a sinus tachycardia, may obtain relief from intravenous then oral beta-blockade. Atenolol 5 mg by slow intravenous injection may be followed by 50 mg orally.[2] The oral dose will achieve peak blood levels by 3–4 hours.

Rarely the pain fails to settle with the conventional approaches and intra-aortic balloon counterpulsation may be necessary, especially if there is associated haemodynamic deterioration or severe ventricular irritability. Angiography with a view to surgery may then be the only option available.

OXYGEN

Arterial hypoxia may occur postinfarction. It makes sense to correct this but no conclusive evidence is available regarding routine oxygen for all patients. I reserve it for patients with cardiac failure, shock, cyanosis or prolonged pain. An oxygenaire safety mask at 81/ minute or medium concentration (MC) mask at 41/minute is used. If there is evidence of chronic lung disease and oxygen is considered essential I would monitor with arterial blood gases and use a 25 per cent mixture.

ANXIETY

See also page 129. It is natural for the patient to feel anxious—the heart has been attacked. It is imperative to provide clear explanations of events and attend to discomfort. If problems continue then diazepam 2–10 mg tds with night sedation (temazepam 10–20 mg) will be effective. I am not in favour of administering daytime benzodiazepines believing that, in the main, the problems they are designed to deal with should be resolved by communication.

DIET

While we can generalize about the type of food that might benefit patients, it is unrealistic in the first few hours to embark on a major change in their dietary habits. The patient feels ill, may be nauseated, and is invariably anorexic. We encourage a simple light diet which is likely to be tolerated. Some will only want a cup of tea, others will manage a bowl of soup and perhaps some chicken or fish. Very few will be able to cope with a heavy meat meal and calorific desserts are unnecessary but if the patient has a favourite food or drink, this should be allowed. Specific dietary advice on obesity can follow later during the ward phase of rehabilitation (see page 129). Diabetes will need careful attention as infarction often upsets control, invariably with hyperglycaemia. A change to subcutaneous insulin or perhaps an infusion of insulin may be needed for even the mildest diabetic whose dietary habits will be upset by the acute illness.

The commode should be used during the stay in the cardiac unit (about 48 hours)

because it is less stressful than the bed pan. Straining at stool should be avoided (Valsalva manoeuvre decreases coronary blood flow) and stool softeners are recommended. Men may stand to urinate.

ANTICOAGULANTS

For the uncomplicated infarct there is no good evidence that routine anticoagulation confers any benefit on mortality. Heparin 5000 units subcutaneously 8 hourly should be used until the patient is mobile to prevent deep venous thrombosis. The incidence of positive leg scans has been reduced by 80 per cent with no increased bleeding.[3]

If embolic complications occur full dose heparinization followed by warfarin therapy should be instituted. Heparin should be given intravenously to prolong the partial thromboplastin time by one and a half to two times (usually 10–15 000 units iv 8 hourly).

Patients with a large anterior infarct and heart failure are at greater risk of systemic embolization and full anticoagulation is recommended, especially if echocardiography identifies extensive left ventricular dysfunction and intracavity thrombus.[4] No evidence exists concerning atrial fibrillation alone but again if this is part of a presentation involving extensive left ventricular dysfunction anticoagulation is recommended.

In contrast to unstable angina the benefits of routine antiplatelet therapy are not yet convincing.[5]

ACTIVITY

Bed rest is recommended for the first 36–48 hours. After this a loosely structured but positive mobilization programme is started (see page 130 and Table 12.1).

In a study evaluating early discharge from hospital it was found that, provided the home environment was suitable, those in a low risk category without complications by the fourth day could safely be discharged after five days

Table 12.1 Hospital mobilization

Uncomplicated infarct

Day	Activity
1–2	Bed rest in cardiac care unit. Use of commode
3–4	General ward. Sit in chair. Use of commode. Walk round bed
5–6	Walk to bathroom. Use of shower. Walking on the ward slowly
7–10	Walking freely on ward. Home possible from day 7. Climb 13 stairs before discharge

Complications

Day	Activity
As needed Cardiac care unit	Bed rest initially then chair in cardiac care unit. Use of commode
Ward 1–2	Walking round bed, commode
3–5	Sit in chair. Walk to bathroom. Walk with assistance
6–10	Walk unassisted. Shower
11–14	Walking freely. Discharge anytime
	Climb stairs before discharge

Patients are usually discharged from Day 8 onwards and should be given a home exercise sheet and the leaflet on coronary heart disease

in hospital.[6] This policy would provide benefits regarding rehabilitation as well as reducing costs. With the addition of beta-blockade as a secondary prevention measure (see page 143) this would provide further safety. Obviously patients with complications must be stabilized and discharged only when mobilized after their intensive therapy. I am therefore in favour of early discharge providing the social environment is satisfactory.

SPECIFIC THERAPY: COMPLICATIONS

Left ventricular failure

The management of heart failure in general is presented in Chapter 17. The most common manifestation of cardiac failure after acute infarction is left ventricular failure. It is imperative to exclude a mechanical cause, especially a ventricular septal defect (VSD) or ruptured papillary muscle leading to severe mitral regurgitation. These are rare (see below) and invariably the problem is left ventricular dysfunction secondary to significant muscle loss.

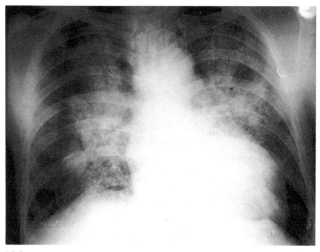

Figure 12.1 Chest x-ray of pulmonary oedema. It is most prominent in the hilar regions (bat's wing appearance).

The diagnosis is based on the symptoms of breathlessness, the clinical findings of basal crackles in the lungs, a III heart sound and sinus tachycardia with the chest x-ray appearances of pulmonary congestion (see Figure 12.1). The signs and symptoms can range from the very mild requiring little or no therapy to the severe requiring intensive haemodynamic support. The most useful clinical classification is that of Killip and Kimball (see Table 12.2).[7] The presence of heart failure is almost universally associated with raised end-diastolic pressures in the left ventricle. The optimal pressure is about 15 mmHg. Below this the chest x-ray will be clear, from 15–18 mmHg the upper zone veins will be filled, from 19–25 mmHg Kerley lines may be visible and above 25 mmHg alveolar oedema will appear. These pressures can be measured by indirect assessment using the pulmonary capillary wedge pressure recorded from right heart catheterization with a Swan-Ganz catheter. Some authorities advocate always using intensive invasive monitoring but this is rarely needed. It is mandatory when heart failure is combined with low arterial pressures but in the vast majority accurate management can be achieved with the minimum intervention and disturbance for the patient. Over-instrumentation can be traumatic.

TREATMENT The patient will be more comfortable sitting up and oxygen should be administered. Diamorphine 5 mg by slow intravenous injection should be given unless recently used for pain relief (within 4 hours).

Opiates are effective by a mixture of systemic venous pooling and actions on the central nervous system.[7]

Diuretics form the mainstay of therapy and should be administered intravenously. As well as promoting diuresis frusemide reduces pulmonary venous pressure by first increasing venous capacitance. The dose is 40–80 mg iv followed by repeat intravenous and then oral therapy depending on effect. Elderly men with prostatic hypertrophy may develop acute retention with the diuresis so 20 mg iv may be a safer initial dose.

Clinical improvement and a fall in pulmonary wedge pressure often precedes the chest x-ray improvement, so if the patient is well a gradual diuresis can then be instituted. This will avoid dehydration and a significant fall in filling pressure which may impair cardiac output (see page 158).

The potassium must be monitored and if oral therapy is instituted potassium replacement considered. Potassium sparing diuretics (eg, spironolactone and amiloride) are more reliable and to be preferred but take two to three days to work. If wheezing is a significant component of the heart failure, aminophylline 250–500 mg by intravenous infusion over 10 minutes may help.

For those with more severe heart failure vasodilators are often necessary. Because of the logic of vasodilatation therapy in heart failure (see page 167) the use of these agents is increasing rapidly so that even in mild failure oral nitrates frequently compliment low dose diuretics. In this way patients may be taking

Class	Status	Mortality per cent
I	No failure clinically	8
II	Crackles at bases. III sound	30
III	Pulmonary oedema	44
IV	Shock	80–100

Table 12.2 Haemodynamic classification (Killip and Kimball)

frusemide 40 mg om, spironolactone 50 mg om and isosorbide 5 mononitrate 20 mg bid, thus avoiding the socially inconvenient and debilitating high dose diuretics. At the point of using intravenous vasodilators it is recommended that pulmonary wedge pressures are monitored to titrate the effect in order to keep the wedge pressure below 20 mmHg but above 15 mmHg. Arterial pressure can be monitored noninvasively if above 90 mmHg but an arterial line will be needed below this. Intravenous vasodilators (invariably nitrates) should be started if the systolic blood pressure is above 100 mmHg and the failure has not responded to intravenous frusemide. Dosage should be titrated against pulmonary wedge pressure and the systolic blood pressure kept above 90 mmHg. Oral mononitrate should start at the same time, pending weaning of intravenous nitrates at a dose of 20 mg bid and occasionally 40 mg bid. It is very rare that other vasodilators are necessary but sodium nitroprusside may be used in addition.

For severe pulmonary oedema where the patient is exhausted, temporary ventilation may allow stabilization and in the acute situation venesection of 1 litre of blood might buy enough time to institute specific therapy. Large pleural effusions should be aspirated immediately.

The role of digoxin is not in doubt where there is atrial fibrillation but raises controversy when there is sinus rhythm. Initial worries that it might increase mortality have been largely dispelled[8] but at best its effects on cardiac output are slight. I would use it in the presence of cardiomegaly and a III sound with a persistent tachycardia in a patient who was not improving on diuretics and vasodilators alone.

Cardiogenic shock

The patient is pale, blood pressure below 90 mmHg systolic, the extremities are cold and clammy and there is oliguria (less than

108

20 cc/hour). The patient may exhibit signs of cerebral hypoperfusion (mental clouding, confusion). The prognosis is poor and here thrombolysis (see page 126) may be a therapeutic option of great importance. These patients undoubtedly consume much time, effort and money for so little long-lasting benefit that inevitably it is sometimes questioned whether it is all in the best interest of the patient.

Before making the diagnosis any agent which might depress left ventricular function should be reversed, eg, beta-blockade reversed by isoprenaline. Cardiogenic shock is confined to those with severe left ventricular pump damage after acute infarction. Arterial and pulmonary lines are essential. Very rarely the patient is hypovolaemic and will respond to an infusion of 500 cc 5 per cent dextrose over 30 minutes. Pain and arrhythmias must be treated and the patient managed in the position he finds most comfortable. Regular monitoring of blood gases is needed to allow for correction of acidosis and a urinary catheter must be inserted to monitor output accurately.

The clinical problem is invariably a low blood pressure combined with a high wedge pressure. The only option is to use inotropic therapy. Dopamine up to 5 µg/kg per minute can be used since above this the vasoconstriction is counterproductive on renal flow and left atrial pressure whereas below this it is beneficial. Dobutamine 2.5–15 µg/kg per minute can be used in addition to dopamine. Dobutamine is less likely than dopamine to increase heart rate, has less adverse or beneficial effects on peripheral vasculature and appears to act directly on cardiac output and reduce pulmonary wedge pressure. By using the combination we get the best of each in a desperate situation. If the pressure then rises a vasodilator such as nitrates may be cautiously introduced to further facilitate cardiac output.

Using intra-aortic balloon counterpulsation seems to buy time at great cost for an inevitable death. When the patient is young and the surgeon willing to try an operation it is difficult to resist. With surgical mortality almost 100 per cent the enthusiasts are now few and far between. This is not the case when there is a mechanical defect such as VSD or where emergency heart transplantation is a realistic option.

I believe the only hope for people with cardiogenic shock rests with trying to open the occluded artery and restore left ventricular function. This means thrombolysis followed by definitive therapy with angioplasty and/or surgery.

Right ventricular infarction

This is usually secondary to inferior infarction. Clinically it should be suspected when the jugular venous pressure (JVP) is raised, the lungs are clear and there is systemic hypotension. Though right ventricular infarction may occur in 25 per cent of cases it inflicts a haemodynamic problem in only 2–5 per cent. It is imperative to carry out echocardiography to exclude pericardial effusion and to look at right ventricular wall movement. In the absence of a classic chest pain/ECG presentation, a massive pulmonary embolus or constrictive pericarditis must be considered in the differential diagnosis.

The treatment is careful volume replacement and as the right ventricle is not contributing to forward flow inotropic support may be necessary. Haemodynamic monitoring is essential during the volume replacement to try to avoid excess replacement (right atrial pressure > 25 mmHg) causing further dilatation of the right ventricle, secondary rise of intrapericardial pressure and a further reduction in left ventricular filling. Though the jugular venous pressure is raised diuretics and vasodilators are contraindicated. These may decrease left ventricular preload and, because the right ventricular infarction is affecting the left ventricle by not providing

preload, this will make the situation worse.

Bradyarrhythmias are common in right ventricular infarction and, as atrial transport is essential, atrioventricular sequential pacing is preferred to ventricular pacing should profound sinus bradycardia or atrioventricular block occur.

Ventricular septal defect

Acute VSDs occur in less than 0.5 per cent of infarcts. Untreated, 95 per cent of patients will die. It usually presents two to ten days postinfarction with a parasternal thrill, right ventricular failure and a new pansystolic murmur at the left sternal edge. Current trends suggest that early operation (within seven days) has a lower overall mortality.[9] Many patients need intra-aortic balloon counterpulsation and inotropic support before surgery and afterwards.

Mitral regurgitation

A harsh systolic murmur radiating to the axilla with sudden haemodynamic deterioration points to acute rupture of a mitral papillary muscle. Usually the sudden volume load in the already affected left ventricle causes acute pulmonary oedema and sometimes shock. Full inotropic support with diuretics, vasodilators and balloon counterpulsation may be needed.

This complication is rare (less than 1 per cent) but in the severe form rapidly fatal with 50 per cent dead in 24 hours. After haemodynamic stabilization (a right heart catheter will have been inserted and oxygen sampling ruled out a VSD) angiography will be done as soon as possible. If the patient is too ill for angiography a mitral valve replacement will be possible using noninvasive echo-Doppler studies to evaluate left ventricular function and mitral pathology. Even the very ill should be able to tolerate coronary angiography if not ventriculography, thus identifying the need for additional bypass surgery.

109

Cardiac rupture

The sudden onset of shock without murmurs three to four days after infarction should raise the question of tamponade secondary to rupture. The patient may cry out before collapsing. An ECG with no output at the onset of a cardiac arrest is also an important sign. If there is time, an echocardiogram will identify pericardial fluid. Otherwise a needle should be advanced to the pericardium and if after aspiration output returns the patient will need immediate surgical repair.

Aneurysms

Ventricular aneurysms may develop within days of the acute infarction. They dilate over the following weeks or months. They present clinically as cardiac failure, ventricular arrhythmias or embolization. The incidence varies from 10 to 20 per cent of acute infarct cases, occurring approximately four times more often on the anteroapical segment of the myocardium than on the inferior wall.[10]

Occasionally a dyskinetic (double beat) apex can be felt but detection of an aneurysm usually follows from noticing persistent ST elevation on the ECG (six weeks postinfarct) and cardiomegaly on x-ray with a boot-shaped appearance (see Figure 12.2). Two-dimensional echocardiography is invaluable in documenting the aneurysm and also for identifying mural thrombus which may be present in up to 50 per cent of cases. The echocardiogram also differentiates false from true aneurysms.[11] Pseudoaneurysms result from rupture of the left ventricle into an area where the pericardium is adherent, thus forming a thin wall. The echo shows pseudoaneurysms having a narrow neck and true aneurysms a wide neck. Pseudoaneurysms may enlarge rapidly and rupture whereas true aneurysms seldom rupture. Pseudoaneurysms should be operated on. True aneurysms should be excluded in those symptomatic on medical treatment. Angiography is essential in all symptomatic cases to document the extent of the aneurysm, the potentially viable residual myocardium (ie, operability) and the presence or absence of additional disease. A recent report of 100 operated cases documented an early mortality of 7 per cent and actuarial survival at five years of 68 per cent.[12] As well as aneurysm resection, mitral valve replacement occurred in eleven cases and bypass surgery in forty. The patient with heart failure is more likely to benefit than the

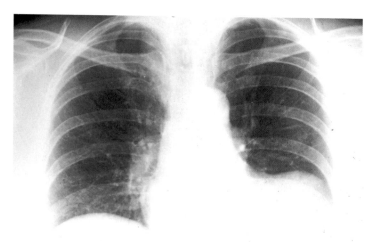

Figure 12.2 Chest x-ray of left ventricular aneurysm. The boot-shaped cardiac silhouette is typical.

patient with ventricular arrhythmias.[13] Improved surgical techniques have therefore led to impressive results in this group and we now need to think of, and exclude, an aneurysm in those incorrectly assumed to have diffuse myocardial disease. An aneurysm without symptoms should be managed medically and patients anticoagulated.

Pericarditis

This may occur early after an infarct (one to five days) or late (three to six weeks) when it is known as Dressler's or the postmyocardial infarction syndrome (see below). Typical pain may occur in 28 per cent of patients with a rub being heard in up to 19 per cent.[14] It is associated with larger infarcts and arrhythmias, especially atrial fibrillation, but not with a higher mortality. Pericardial effusions that are significant are, however, rare and not worsened by anticoagulants so that, if needed, anticoagulation is not contraindicated when pericarditis complicates acute infarction.[15] Treatment is effective with indomethacin 25–50 mg 8 hourly or aspirin 600 mg 6 hourly.

Dressler's syndrome

Pleuropericardial pain and fever, a rub and pericardial and/or pleural effusions are the hallmarks of Dressler's syndrome.[16] Some or all of these features may be present, with a presentation typically in the first three months after infarction. The erythrocyte sedimentation rate (ESR) and white count are often raised and heart-reactive antibodies detected. It is important to separate this benign self-limiting illness from infarct extension and pulmonary embolism.

Treatment is symptomatic as for pericarditis. In severe cases steroids may be necessary, though relapses may occur on cessation of therapy so gradual withdrawal is advised.[17] Rarely Dressler's syndrome can develop into a recurring illness similar to benign relapsing pericarditis. The ESR can be useful for monitoring response to therapy.

Infarct extention

This is believed to occur in 20 per cent of patients within five days of an infarct[18] but this incidence is likely to decrease with the widespread use of drug therapy in the early phases of care (eg, nitrates and beta-blockers). Pericarditis may be confused with infarct extension or be a part of it. Management of an infarct extension is as for the original event.

Hypertension

If after relief of pain and anxiety hypertension remains (blood pressure > 160/95 mmHg) treatment should be started based on the haemodynamic status of the patient. Dietary advice will be necessary but in the short term beta-blockade, diuretics and calcium antagonists are initiated as appropriate (eg, if no failure give atenolol 50 mg daily, if bronchospasm but no failure use a calcium antagonist, if failure use a diuretic and possibly a vasodilator later).

Arrhythmias

This is not a book about the fine details of arrhythmia detection, but it is concerned with the practical aspects of identification and treatment. Many books dedicated to arrhythmias exist and in the Appendix a list of recommended reading will be found.

Ventricular arrhythmias

Here we are concerned with ventricular arrhythmias at the time of acute infarction. Chronic arrhythmias are discussed in Chapter 19 (page 185). Ventricular fibrillation is discussed in the context of resuscitation (see page 97).

PROPHYLAXIS

Lignocaine

The most dangerous time for ventricular fibrillation is the first hour when 40 per cent of deaths occur. This has reinforced the argument for lignocaine 300 or 400 mg im in the pre-hospital phase (see page 93). By the time the patients reach hospital we are already seeing the survivors, but even in these there is an incidence of ventricular fibrillation in up to 10 per cent in the cardiac care unit.

'Warning arrhythmias'—extrasystoles greater than six per minute of multifocal origins, runs or couplets—were considered likely early signs of ventricular fibrillation.[19] However, detailed study showed that ventricular fibrillation could develop in 40 per cent without any warning.[20] R-on-T extrasystoles are considered more threatening because they often precede ventricular fibrillation or ventricular tachycardia. This has led to the proposal that all suitable patients should have a prophylactic infusion of lignocaine after hospital arrival.[21] The problem is one of balance.[22] Given that the hospital incidence of ventricular fibrillation is low and that the unit should be able to respond immediately to ventricular fibrillation, are the potential side-effects of the regime (risk) worth the benefit? I believe not. A simple regime is possible (bolus of 100 mg, 4 mg/minute for 1 hour, 2 mg/minute for 24 hours) but there is the potential for side-effects (nausea, numbness, confusion, respiratory depression, convulsions, bradycardia, sinus arrest, heart block and hypotension) which are blood level dependent. These can occur even with the simplest regime because of variable hepatic metabolism and hepatic blood flow, which may be reduced in heart failure. Therefore I would not use lignocaine prophylactically unless R-on-T ectopics were identified.

There is no evidence that longterm antiarrhythmic therapy after primary ventricular fibrillation is prophylactic against further events.[23] Here persistent arrhythmias postinfarction may be a marker of adverse prognosis and suggest the need for a thorough invasive and noninvasive assessment rather than symptomatic oral antiarrythmics alone.

Intravenous beta-blockade

Intravenous beta-blockade (metoprolol) has been proved to prevent ventricular fibrillation.[24] It is known that acute infarction is associated with catecholamine release, with the potential for increasing oxygen demand and promoting ventricular irritability. A study of intravenous atenolol[25] showed a significant reduction in ventricular arrhythmias. Combining hospital mortality with patients resuscitated from ventricular fibrillation and discharged alive gave a significant result in favour of atenolol. This, however, was a study of only 182 patients. The same group coordinated a multicentre study involving 16 027 patients using atenolol for early intervention.[26] The mortality data are shown in Table 12.3. Atenolol was administered 5–10 mg iv followed by 100 mg oral daily for seven days. It is obvious that the benefits are in the early group. Infarction is known to be usually over by 4 hours and the risks occur before this, so a case can be made for early use of intravenous atenolol or other beta-blockers. The reduction in mortality is calculated at 30 per cent, equivalent to one life saved per 150 patients treated. There were no other adverse effects of note, no doubt because of careful patient selection.

Placed in the practical context:

1   There is a reasonable argument for lignocaine 300–400 mg im pre-hospital providing there is no bradycardia or shock or access to a defibrillator (see page 93).
2   There is no support for routine prophylactic lignocaine after arrival at hospital.
3   Intravenous beta-blockade is indicated in the first 4 hours if no contraindications exist.
4   Outside these groups treatment should be based on events, ie, lignocaine for arrhythmias and beta-blockers for pain or arrhythmias.
5   If beta-blockade is given intravenously it should be continued orally.[27]

TREATMENT OF VENTRICULAR EXTRASYSTOLES

When a decision to treat ventricular extrasystoles has been made first

1 Check the patient is not in pain—this can be a cause.
2 Check for hypokalaemia—correct it intravenously.
3 Administer oxygen.

If there are still R-on-T ectopics (see Figure 12.3) or rapidly increasing numbers, lignocaine should be administered iv 100 mg bolus, 4 mg/minute for 1 hour then 2 mg/minute. If this is not successful a further bolus should be given of 50 mg and then a further 50 mg. Simply increasing the rate of infusion is not effective because of the long time needed to obtain a new steady state level.

If unsuccessful and there are haemodynamic problems from the arrhythmias, I try procainamide 100 mg iv/minute to 1 g followed by an infusion of 2 mg/minute. An alternative is amiodarone 300 mg iv. I continue infusions for at least 24 hours.

VENTRICULAR TACHYCARDIA

This is defined as three or more consecutive ventricular extrasystoles (see Figure 12.4). It may be brief or sustained. If brief lignocaine is given as for extrasystoles,[28] if sustained and symptomatic a dc shock is necessary. If the ventricular tachycardia is resistant to lignocaine, procainamide and/or amiodarone should be tried. In rare instances, control can be achieved only with the help of balloon counterpulsation and/or overdrive pacing buying time for conventional antiarrhythmics to establish control.

There is often debate as to whether a ventricular tachycardia is really ventricular tachycardia or supraventricular tachyarrhythmia with aberrant conduction.[29] By far the commonest after infarction is ventricular tachycardia *even if* there is no haemodynamic upset.

Differentiating between supraventricular tachyarrhythmia and ventricular tachycardia

(i) If it is irregular, consider atrial fibrillation with bundle branch block (see Figure 12.5).

Days from randomization	Atenolol	Control	p
0–1*	119	171	< 0.002
2–3	89	90	NS
4–7	104	103	NS
Subtotal 8–365+	665	694	NS
Total	977	1058	< 0.03

Table 12.3 ISIS mortality data. Deaths (vascular) no.

* Period of greatest risk. NS=Not significant.

(ii) Is there evidence of atrioventricular dissociation?—Ventricular tachycardia.

(iii) If there is a normal QRS in sinus rhythm, is QRS width now > 140 ms?—Ventricular tachycardia.

(iv) Is the tachycardia like a previous ventricular extrasystole?—Ventricular tachycardia.

(v) Does carotid sinus massage cause slowing?—Supraventricular tachyarrhythmia (no effect is unhelpful).

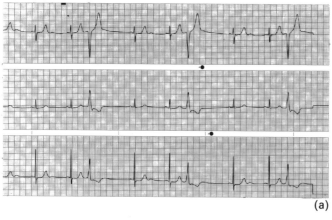

(a)

Figure 12.3 Ventricular extrasystoles.
(a) Unifocal: simultaneous three-channel trace: note, the broad QRS complex, no preceding P wave and compensatory pause. A twelve-lead ECG will reveal a bizarre axis.
(b) Multifocal: two different shaped extrasystoles indicating different origins.
(c) R-on-T: triggers a three-beat run of ventricular tachycardia.
(d) Bigeminy: one extrasystole follows each sinus beat. Consider digoxin toxicity.

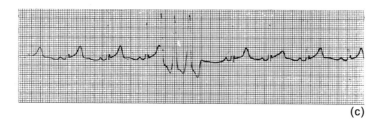

(b)

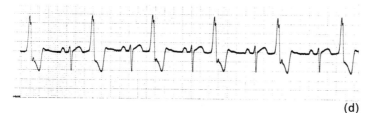

(c)

(d)

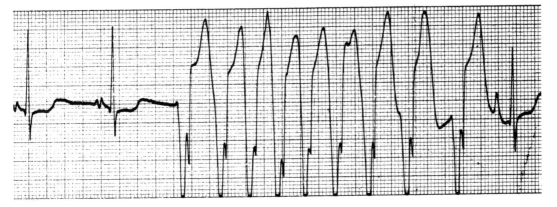

Figure 12.4 Ventricular tachycardia.

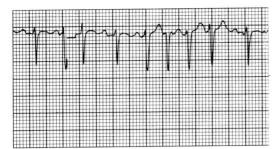

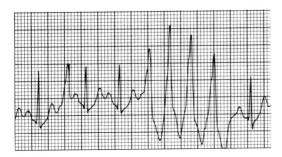

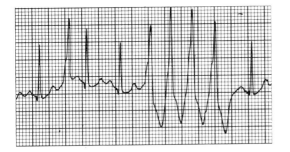

Figure 12.5 Three-channel trace simultaneously identifies paroxysmal atrial fibrillation rather than ventricular tachycardia. Top trace clarifies.

(vi) Is there ventricular concordance (see Figure 12.6)?—Ventricular tachycardia. This means uniform positive or negative deflections V1–V6.

If there is still doubt treatment is as follows:

(i) Record a twelve-lead ECG—check the above.
(ii) If haemodynamic problems—dc shock—record twelve-lead in sinus rhythm and compare with tachycardia for further therapy.
(iii) Amiodarone intravenously will deal with both.

IDIOVENTRICULAR RHYTHM

Idioventricular tachycardia is benign and rarely needs treating. This is a ventricular tachycardia with a slow rate, usually less than 120 beats/minute. It is invariably associated with acute infarction, when its presence in the absence of conventional ECG changes should raise the suspicion of infarction. Typically there are runs of up to fifteen or so broad QRS complexes at a rate less than 100 beats/ minute. Fusion beats may be present (see Figure 12.7).

TORSADE DE POINTES

This is ventricular tachycardia with a rotating axis (see Figure 12.8).[30] It is associated with a long QT interval on the ECG. It can be caused by hypokalaemia, hypomagnesaemia and conventional antiarrhythmic drugs such as lignocaine, mexiletene and disopyramide. Treatment surrounds correcting the electrolytes,

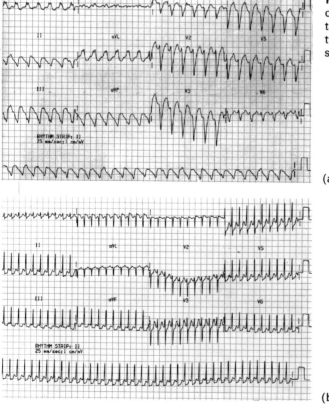

Figure 12.6 (a) Ventricular concordance of ventricular tachycardia contrasts with (b) twelve-lead ECG of supraventricular tachycardia.

(a)

(b)

avoiding the pro-arrhythmic drugs and if necessary inserting a pacemaker to overdrive the tachycardia. Beta-blockade may be helpful in addition.[31]

ATRIAL ARRHYTHMIAS

Atrial extrasystoles

The incidence is about 30 per cent.[32] By themselves these are usually benign but when present frequently they may precede atrial flutter or fibrillation. They are common with pericarditis. The impulse originates from an ectopic focus in the atria so that the P wave related to the extrasystoles is different from the sinus rhythm P wave. The QRS complex is usually narrow and similar to the normal sinus complex. The compensatory pause after the extrasystole is incomplete. Comparing atrial extrasystoles (see Figure 12.9) with ven-

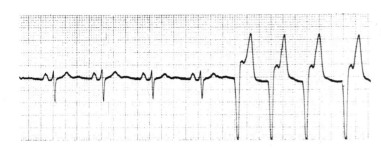

Figure 12.7 Idioventricular rhythm.

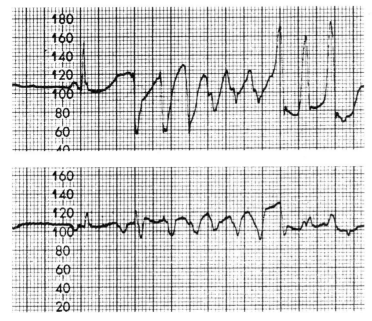

Figure 12.8 Torsade de pointes.

tricular (see Figure 12.3) the width of the QRS complex and P wave relationship and measuring the compensatory pause usually identifies which is which. Monitor traces may not be clear so a V1 on the ECG should be taken to identify the P wave.

Treatment is not necessary if they are occasional but frequent atrial extrasystoles should be suppressed with intravenous beta-blockade or digoxin to prevent atrial fibrillation occurring with a rapid ventricular response which may exacerbate the ischaemia.

Sinus tachycardia

This is a regular sinus rhythm of over 100 beats/minute. It should be thought of as a marker of pain, anxiety, fever or heart failure and appropriate therapy administered. Sometimes it is inappropriate, ie, there is no obvious cause, when it settles quickly with beta-blockade.

Atrial fibrillation

Sustained atrial fibrillation affects about 10 per cent post acute infarction.[32] The rapid ventricular response and the loss of the P waves' contribution to cardiac output may cause severe hypotension, heart failure or even extension of the infarct. It is recognized (see Figure 12.10) by chaotic atrial activity with no P waves but rapid irregular fibrillating waves (about 400–600 beats/minute). The atrioventricular node can only conduct up to 200 beats/minute so an irregular ventricular response occurs depending on the impulses being handled at the atrioventricular node. The QRS complex is usually narrow but atrial fibrillation may be associated with either right or left bundle branch block.

Nurses should always record the apex rate. If the fibrillation is associated with haemodynamic deterioration a prompt synchronized dc shock should be given (100 joules, increas-

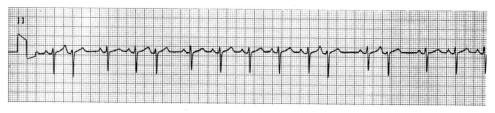

Figure 12.9 Atrial extrasystoles. Note the similarity between the extrasystole and sinus beats. Contrast with Figure 12.3a.

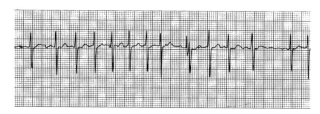

Figure 12.10 Atrial fibrillation.

ing as necessary). If pericarditis is present this should be treated but the likelihood of a relapse is high when pericarditis is present. When there is no haemodynamic problem and after a dc shock the patient should be digitalized. Further slowing of the rate can be achieved with beta-blockade or verapamil but if failure has been a problem these drugs should be avoided and digoxin used, with amiodarone if digoxin alone is not fully effective. The drugs can be withdrawn in most cases five to six days after the acute episode but reinstated if there is a relapse.

Atrial flutter

This is uncommon—about 1–2 per cent. There is no P wave but a re-entry mechanism leads to an atrial rate of 300 beats/minute. The atrioventricular block is a function of 300, the commonest being 2:1, ie, the ventricular rate is 150 beats/minute. The classical 'saw tooth' or 'picket fence' flutter waves are

shown in Figure 12.11—these can be revealed best when carotid massage increases the atrioventricular block leading to a variable ventricular rate. The QRS is usually narrow and the rhythm best detected in leads II, III, aVf and V1. Treatment is as for atrial fibrillation but dc conversion is likely to be successful as low as 50 joules.

Supraventricular tachycardia

This is usually the result of re-entry within the atrioventricular node leading to a heart rate of 150–220 beats/minute. Because of this mechanism it is unlikely to present for the first time at acute infarction. The tachycardia is invariably flutter with 2:1 block.

P waves may be visible before, during or after the QRS complex depending upon the sequence of activation. The QRS may be narrow or aberrant if, for example, bundle branch block occurs (see Figure 12.12).

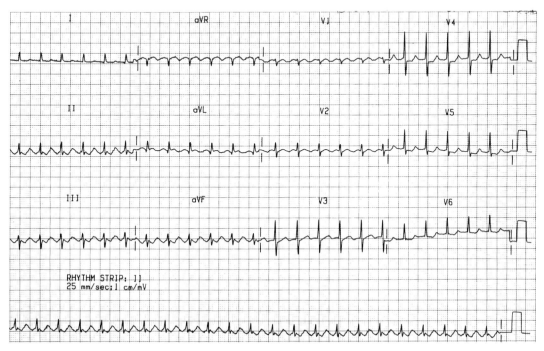

Figure 12.11 Atrial flutter.

119

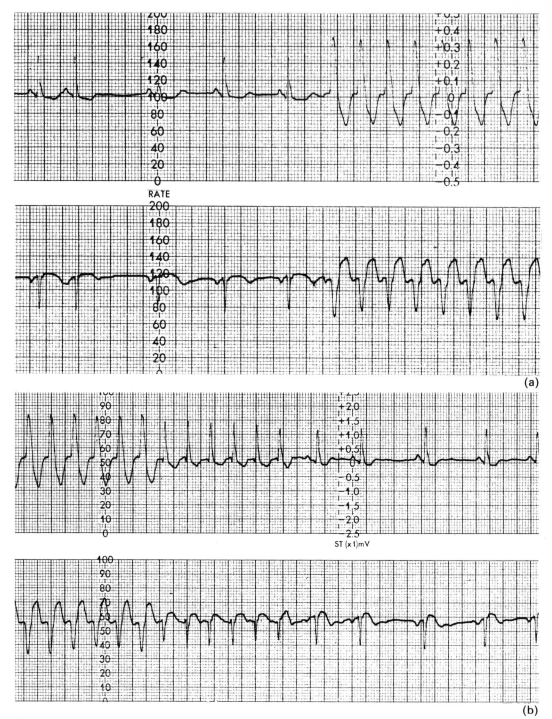

Figure 12.12 Simultaneous two-channel traces: Supraventricular tachycardia. (a) Onset is related to a P wave, QRS width less than 140 ms. (b) Termination shows transient loss of bundle branch block before sinus rhythm is restored.

Carotid sinus massage may terminate the attack. If haemodynamic problems exist dc shock is necessary. If there are no haemodynamic problems verapamil 5–10 mg iv is highly effective but it should not be used with digoxin or beta-blockade for fear of inducing asystole. I personally prefer intravenous beta-blockade because of the additional anti-ischaemic effects and the possibility of combining it with digoxin both intravenously and orally should the rhythm relapse.

Junctional rhythm

This is more common after inferior infarction. The junctional area takes over as the pacemaker because of sinus bradycardia (ie, the junction is faster). The P waves usually are buried in the QRS or follow it (see Figure 12.13). Treatment should be withheld if there is no problem (the slow rate may be beneficial) but if a fall in blood pressure or cardiac output occurs, atropine (0.3 mg increased to 2.4 mg iv) should be tried with temporary pacing if ineffective. Atropine may need to be repeated.

Atrioventricular block

Here there is a major difference between inferior infarction and anterior infarction. Atrioventricular node block is more frequent with inferior infarction due to the blood supply arising in 90 per cent of cases from the right coronary artery, which is the usual vessel occluded.[33] For anterior infarction to inflict damage in the conducting system there is usually substantial muscle loss and a poor prognosis. The differences are summarized in Table 12.4.

First degree atrioventricular block

The PR interval is greater than 0.2 seconds. The rhythm is regular and ventricular depolarization is achieved normally apart from delay in the atrioventricular node (see Figure 12.14). It needs no specific therapy but agents that depress the conducting system should be avoided (eg, beta-blockers, verapamil, digoxin).

Second degree atrioventricular block

WENCKEBACH OR MOBITZ TYPE I   There is gradual prolongation of the PR interval as the atrioventricular node becomes increasingly refractory and then conduction fails (see Figure 12.15a). The block is at nodal level. It usually follows inferior infarction. It requires watching and in 80 per cent of cases no specific therapy. Occasionally it progresses and pacemaker intervention is required. (It may respond to atropine.)

MOBITZ TYPE II   There is now intermittent failure of conduction and beats are dropped. The PR interval is usually normal and suddenly the P wave is not followed by a QRS complex (see Figure 12.15b). The number of P waves to QRS results in the terminology 2:1, 3:1 etc, block. The more narrow the QRS the higher the block (the wider the QRS the lower the block, suggesting more extensive damage, especially in the presence of anterior infarction).

I advocate temporary pacing in this situation because the rhythm is much more volatile. Until pacing is established atropine and isoprenaline can be tried if the rate is slow and the output reduced but these drugs are not substitutes—they are a holding manoeuvre.

Third degree atrioventricular block (complete block)

The onset may be sudden or progressive. After anterior infarction it usually represents severe muscle loss. With inferior infarction the block is nodal and a junctional (narrow QRS) pacemaker takes over with an escape rate of forty to sixty beats/minute. There is no relationship between the P and QRS (see Figure 12.16). With anterior infarction the block is at His Purkinje level, the escape rhythm unreliable and of the order at best of twenty to forty beats/minute. Again there is no connection between P and QRS but the QRS now has a broad complex.

If the rate is good after inferior infarction a conservative approach can be tried using atropine for temporary slowing. However, if hae-

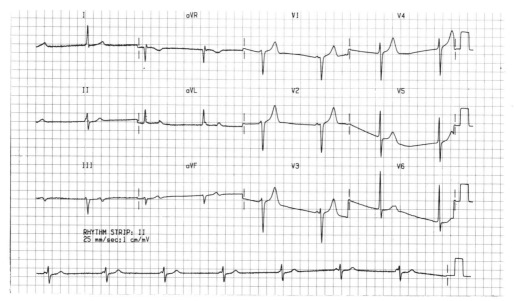

Figure 12.13 Junctional escape rhythm. When the sinus node fails the inherent automaticity of conducting tissue below the sinus node assumes pacemaker function. Here the P waves can be seen to be slower than the QRS complexes which are narrow because the ventricle is depolarized by normal pathways.

	Inferior infarction	Anterior infarction
Incidence	5–10 per cent	1–3 per cent
Location	AV node	His-Purkinje system
Morality	20–40 per cent	70–80 per cent
Common abnormalities	First degree, Mobitz I	Mobitz II
Complete block	AV node, narrow QRS. Rate 40–60	Below AV node, wide QRS. Rate 20–40
Haemodynamic upset	Occasional	Frequent

Table 12.4 Site of infarction and atrioventricular (AV) block

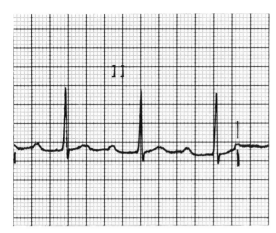

Figure 12.14 First degree atrioventricular block.

modynamic problems occur or if the rate is varying considerably, a temporary pacemaker is needed. After anterior infarction a temporary pacemaker is always needed.

If anxious I advocate pacing. If there is an acute presentation on Friday evening I advocate pacing. In short I would put a temporary pacing wire in if I had any doubts about progress.

Atrioventricular dissociation

The atrial rate is lower than the ventricular rate. The P waves can be 'marched through' the QRS. No specific therapy is needed if the ventricular rate is adequate.

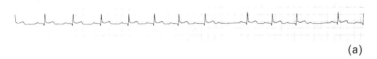

(a)

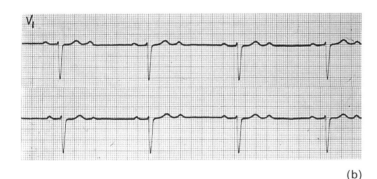

(b)

Figure 12.15 (a) Wenckebach or Mobitz type I second degree atrioventricular block. The atrioventricular node is increasingly refractory until failure of conduction occurs. The PR interval is seen to lengthen before conduction failure. The QRS is narrow as ventricular depolarization is by normal pathways. (b) Mobitz type II. The PR interval is constant but there is intermittent failure of atrioventricular conduction.

BUNDLE BRANCH BLOCK

After acute infarction new bundle branch block is associated with an increased risk of Mobitz type II and complete block—about 20 per cent.[34] Old bilateral bundle branch block and infarction does not carry the same risk of progression as new bilateral bundle branch block—10 per cent compared with 35 per cent. Bilateral bundle branch block refers to alternating right bundle branch block and LBBB, or right bundle branch block with left anterior or posterior hemiblock. A prophylactic pacemaker is indicated because ventricular standstill may occur abruptly with new bila-

teral bundle branch block, but it is not necessary with new isolated right bundle branch block or LBBB unless there is a new development of first degree heart block. Careful monitoring is essential. Selective ECGs are shown in Figures 12.17–12.19.

PERMANENT PACING

I allow infarcts two weeks to recover normal conduction. I also tape the rhythm for 24 hours when mobile and do an exercise ECG before discharge. I insert a permanent pacemaker if there is any residual problem documented on these tests or if full recovery does

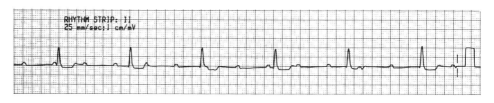

Figure 12.16 Complete heart block. There is no correlation between the P waves and QRS complexes.

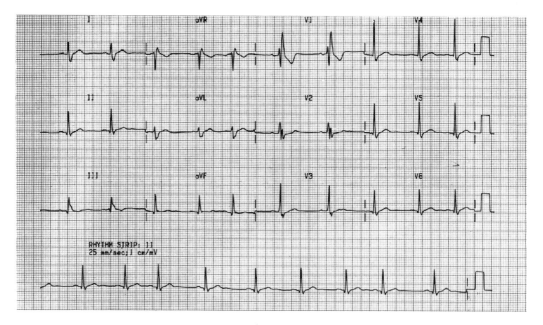

Figure 12.17 Right bundle branch block. Large R wave in VI, deep S in I and V6. QRS > 0.12 ms.

124

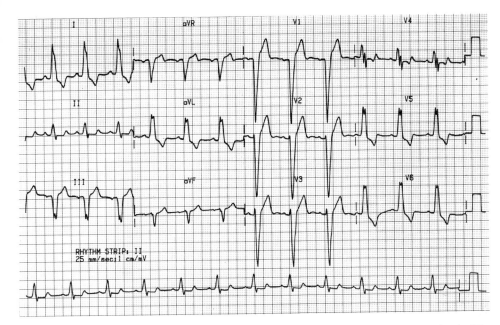

Figure 12.18 Left bundle branch block. Wide QRS positive in I and V6, negative in V1.

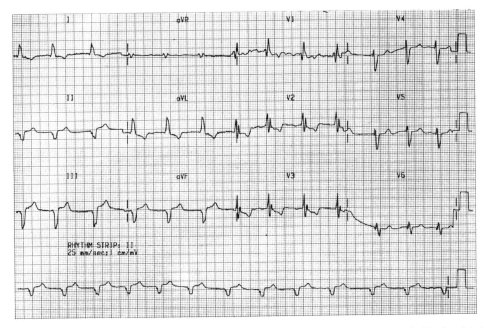

Figure 12.19 Bifascicular block with atrial fibrillation. Right bundle branch block with left anterior hemiblock. Left axis deviation. High risk of complete block in acute infarction.

not occur. Evidence of bifascicular block with symptoms merits pacing. I have the impression that the elderly require pacing more frequently after infarction complicated by heart block. If I have doubts I insert a permanent system.

THROMBOLYSIS

At the time of writing, this is the most active area of infarct management. Thrombolytic agents are the subject of intensive investigation because of the potential to reverse the arterial thrombosis that has initiated myocardial infarction. Intracoronary infusion of streptokinase restores patency within 2–3 hours in 84 per cent.[35] The intracoronary route, however, demands a catheter laboratory to be available and takes time and specialized manpower. Time is precious, for it appears that to prevent myocardial loss recanalization must be within 2–3 hours.[35] In practice therefore most effort has to be directed at the intravenous route.

Streptokinase, which is widely available, has the potential disadvantages of being antigenic and inducing a diffuse fibrinolytic state for over 24 hours. Relatively fibrin-specific agents have been developed to circumvent these problems and include tissue type plasminogen activator (rTPA) prourokinase and acylated streptokinase plasminogen complex (ASPAC). For the time being only streptokinase is widely available and the intravenous dose appears to be 1 million units given over 30 minutes. In the largest intravenous study (GISSI)[37] there was an 18 per cent reduction in fatality, with the greatest benefit below 3 hours and over 50 per cent reduction within 1 hour.

How do these observations translate to current clinical practice?

1 In apparently hopeless cases arriving within 6 hours, ie, those in cardiogenic shock, there is little to be lost and an enormous potential gain.

2 Streptokinase intracoronary is effective in recanalization so in suitable cases this should be considered within 2–3 hours.[36]

3 The left ventricle appears savable only at 2–3 hours, so recanalization after this will be unlikely to produce benefit.

4 The intravenous option is available to all and recanalization rates are reasonable— of the order of 50–60 per cent.[38]

5 Recanalization does not remove an underlying significant stenosis and definitive therapy to that by percutaneous transluminal coronary angioplasty or surgery should follow; ie, thrombolysis is a holding manoeuvre.

6 Reperfusion can be measured by ventricular arrhythmias (prophylactic lignocaine is routine) and an early CPK rise at about 15 hours.[39]

7 Those with recent operations or peptic ulcers or cerebrovascular episodes present contraindications.

8 To avoid antigenic effects give hydrocortisone 100 mg iv.

9 To avoid spasm start intravenous nitrates and continue for 48 hours.

10 Additional anticoagulation with heparin is routine but not logically defined.

I would suggest the plan as shown opposite.

The future for the relatively fibrin-specific agents is exciting but the potential for reversing infarction will demand a greatly increased educational programme. The patient (and doctor) must recognize the problem early enough. Finally if the efforts of the investigators confirm the effectiveness of thrombolysis in its safer form, eg, rTPA,[40] the implications for angiography and surgery are enormous. Furthermore we can conceive its use for out of hospital (family doctor, in ambulances). In the interest of the patient let us hope the optimism will translate into practical reality.[41]

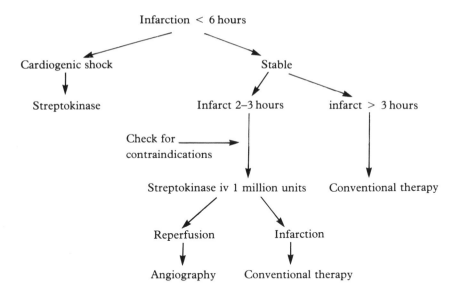

Infarction < 6 hours

Cardiogenic shock   Stable

Streptokinase   Infarct 2–3 hours   infarct > 3 hours

Check for
contraindications

Streptokinase iv 1 million units   Conventional therapy

Reperfusion   Infarction

Angiography   Conventional therapy

PRACTICAL POINTS

- Relief of pain is essential. Ask patients frequently; they often suffer in silence.

- Oxygen is not routine but may help in heart failure.

- Anxiety responds to explanation and pain relief.

- Subcutaneous heparin is used to prevent deep venous thrombosis.

- Average hospital stay is 8–10 days with rapid mobilization.

- Cardiac care units optimize trained staff and deal with complications.

- Cardiogenic shock is invariably fatal but thrombolysis and angioplasty offer new hope.

- Pericarditis occurs in nearly one-third of patients and responds to indomethacin.

- Prompt attention to arrhythmias may save life as the period of electrical instability is usually short.

- Thrombolysis and angioplasty are likely to increase as forms of immediate therapy, though the ventricle is irreversibly lost if deprived of blood for over 3–4 hours.

13
Rehabilitation

BACKGROUND

Rehabilitation is concerned with restoring disabled people as quickly and as sensibly as possible to a full physical, social and mental level of activity. This assumes that a level of activity, which the doctor or multidisciplinary team felt acceptable, existed before the illness. This is not always the case, nor is it always the wish of an individual to be more active than before or to live a different life after an illness. Health care teams involved in rehabilitation set ideal standards of activity which are conditioned in many ways by their own levels of activity and, by definition, people actively involved in rehabilitation are most unlikely to be inactive. Yet many members of the community are quite happy leading a sedentary existence, exerting the minimum effort and enjoying watching television and social drinking. The problem to be faced in rehabilitation is restoring the person to where he was before the illness and convincing the patient that by making various lifestyle changes a further illness may be prevented. As the personality of each patient is so different, objectives must always be adjusted to the individual. Over-zealousness will be met in some with a vigorous and positive response but others will default and be lost to the efforts of secondary prevention.[1,2]

THE HEART

Being the organ most associated with emotion it is subconsciously felt to be the most vulnerable. When illness strikes the heart the emotional responses can exacerbate the problem, and no more so than in the situation of myocardial infarction.

MYOCARDIAL INFARCTION

Rehabilitation begins at the onset of the illness with as much communication as possible between the patient, spouse and family. The outcome will be related to personality (coping ability and comprehension of the illness), social background (work, housing, finances, responsibilities to family and theirs to the patient) and family strengths and weaknesses (married, divorced, strength of spouse).

Normal reactions to an infarct are denial, anxiety and depression. The degree of the reactions is usually mild from 'Why me?', 'Can't be', to a temporary bout of 'the blues'. Occasionally the reaction is pathological, invariably because of a preceding problem whether recognized or not, and profound depression or rarely a psychotic episode, may follow. Emotional disturbances can be expected in about 60 per cent of people admitted to a cardiac care unit.

The onset of myocardial infarction is painful and frightening. In many ways how the patient copes depends on how he is dealt with initially. The immediate relief of pain with intravenous diamorphine with the antiemetic cyclizine helps the patient and family's immediate fears which revolve around death. The family unit is relieved to be in a 'safe' environment (hospital) and the immediate alleviation of the major symptom reinforces in its members the idea that whatever has or is happening, the patient is 'in the right hands'.

CARDIAC CARE UNIT

Initially the patient is anxious, tired and may still be in pain (see Table 13.1). At this point the diagnosis should be explained in simple terms to both the patient and spouse at the same interview so that they are equally well-informed. I tell the patient that the heart is bruised and sore and needs to rest, and the best way he can help himself for the first day is by resting in bed; I try to communicate to the patient even at this stage that he is helping himself also. The monitors and gadgets are explained as routine protection to try to give an impression of a team approach, with the patient being the most important individual in the team.

Common problems

DENIAL This is common, especially with professional people—particularly doctors.

Denial usually gives way to reality but often in the type A personality (aggressive, ambitious, impatient) it persists, and though this may be useful in the short term with regard to a positive approach to recovery, in the long term it may be detrimental. It is estimated that 20 per cent of people who have sustained an infarct still doubt that it happened after two weeks. Men exhibit more denial than women and it is invariably men who take their own discharge against advice.

ANXIETY This is a universal problem—'What is wrong with me? Am I going to die?' Deaths of others occur in the unit and then the 'umbilical cord' is severed as the patient is transferred to a general ward. At this point more questions will arise; patients must have the opportunity to ask them and receive answers. The doctor or nurse must sit on the bed and look at the patient, not talk down to him from the standing position. Patients with limited intelligence need more patience, not less time. Moving to the ward is accompanied by stating how pleased you are with the patient's progress. The patient and family are more able to understand the meaning of the illness and plan for the future:

- Two weeks—in hospital for healing and gradual mobilization.
- Two weeks—at home very gradually increasing activity.
- Two weeks—at home accelerating back to normal with a positive approach to the future and a six-week medical assessment where practitioners can either deal with problems or send the patient back to work.

Of course this is simple, but keeping it simple and straightforward is the key to recovery. Those who remain anxious may benefit from a short course of diazepam but it is best to try to avoid this at all costs.

Table 13.1 Patients' thoughts

What is wrong with me?

Am I going to die?

How can I stop this happening again?

Why can my children not visit?

I am bored in hospital.

I am lonely at night.

Why is my wife/husband so anxious?

What about my job?

Should I cancel my holiday?

DEPRESSION Patients may not experience this problem but if they do it usually presents on the third day after leaving the cardiac care unit. Concern over jobs in the current economic climate, especially for heavy goods vehicle or public service vehicle drivers, and guilt, invariably because of heavy smoking and helplessness, are paramount. The male patient feels his 'manhood' is challenged—especially the younger man. With a positive approach to the future this is less of a problem. Directing the patient towards the future and planning the rehabilitation circumvents many of the problems without recourse to specific antidepressant therapy. If, however, depression persists, psychiatric assessment should be arranged before prescribing drugs because there may have been a preceding problem which needs specialist evaluation.

BOOKLETS

No matter how clearly the doctor and nurse feels they have expressed themselves, the patient and family, on the background of stress and anxiety, misinterpret or become confused by the information given. Providing written information for the patient and spouse as soon as possible answers many of the raised and unraised questions which preoccupy all concerned. In a study I carried out a far greater understanding of the illness and a more satisfactory recovery was found in those given written as well as oral information. Booklets are not a substitute for talking, but complement and often enhance the interviews by prompting the patient to ask awkward and relevant questions.[3]

THE GENERAL WARD

While this is a sign of progress it is also the time to begin the first aspects of physical rehabilitation. An attempt has been made to allay the anxieties of the patient and family and a positive move forward should now

130

begin. Our own rehabilitation programme at Lewisham Hospital in London is now run by highly trained, sensitive and thoughtful physiotherapists. Where necessary, patients with difficulties can be seen by a psychiatrist who may enrol them in a group counselling session where concerns can be freely discussed and mutual reassurance given.

The importance of education must be emphasized, as this will alleviate fear and anxiety. If the doctor really does not have time to talk he should say so but emphatically make the point that he is going to come back. Simple repetitive information is all that is needed. From the general ward and into convalescence, recommendations on management and prevention must be given to the patient. Our inpatient programme is illustrated in Table 12.1.

AFTER DISCHARGE

The hospital environment is controlled and protective, and naturally anxiety occurs when the patient is discharged. Feelings of fatigue usually follow the environmental change but can also reflect too much physical activity. The patient should be told to anticipate this and to be sure to rest and get a good night's sleep. If this proves difficult, night sedation should be ordered from the family doctor. Aches and pains previously discounted now assume greater importance but they are invariably sharp and positional and not cardiac. The patient should be told the difference between cardiac and non-cardiac pain.

Getting back to normal
The days of prolonged rest and convalescence are over except for those who have sustained massive infarcts with substantial left ventricular damage. Early ambulation avoids physical problems such as deep venous thrombosis as well as psychological problems such as anxiety and depression.[4]

Physical activity

Physical activity programmes have not been shown to lengthen life or reduce subsequent cardiac events. They need to be tailored to the individual. If a satisfactory programme is adopted, a subsequent increase in the sense of well-being and decreased anxiety follows. By exercising in a programme with others the group atmosphere is encouraged, opportunities for communication fostered and the sense of isolation and guilt diminished. Our initial home programme is shown in Table 13.2 and our gymnasium programme in Table 13.3. Following on from this our patients have continued exercises at home and formed a once weekly coronary club. It is very rare for cardiac arrests to occur in a properly directed and supervised programme with individual prescriptions but we have full resuscitation facilities on site.[5]

Treadmill ECG

All our patients under sixty-five of age who have sustained an uncomplicated myocardial infarct undergo routine treadmill exercise testing to their maximal ability within two to six weeks of their infarct. It has been shown that those with a positive test have an increased morbidity and mortality at one year and that elective bypass surgery may be able to prevent subsequent infarction and death.[6] In addition, by combining the treadmill test with the rehabilitation process, we have been able to reinforce the recovery of the patient as well as to emphasize our continuing commitment to his care and progress.

Sexual activity

Early studies reported a marked increase in heart rate in men and women at the time of orgasm, with increases of over 100 beats/minute with significant increases in respiratory rate and blood pressure. However, these were all in young volunteers in an unnatural environment and involved relationships with strangers.[7,8]

Fortunately, several studies are now available which look at a more representative sector of the population, and these can be used as a basis for initiating advice and guidelines to cardiac patients.[9] Importantly, these studies involved married couples and were conducted in the home (familiar) environment.

The average resting heart rate was 60 ± 8 beats/minute rising to 92 ± 13 at intromission and achieving a maximal rate of 114 ± 14 at orgasm. At 120 seconds of resolution the rate had already fallen to 69 ± 12 beats/minute. Similar responses occurred whether the man was on top or underneath. Blood pressure rose from a mean of 112/66 mmHg at rest to 148/79 at intromission and a maximum of 163/81 at orgasm. Resting levels were achieved 120 seconds into resolution. Position again made no significant difference.

An evaluation of middle-aged (forty-seven years) patients with ischaemic heart disease recorded an average maximal heart rate of 117 beats/minute (range 90–144) during sex, compared with 120 (range 107–130) during other activities.[10,11] In six the maximal heart rate during sexual intercourse was greater than that during work and in eight it was less. While most studies have taken place in the USA, similar findings were reported in patients with angina pectoris who were studied in the UK, with heart rates during sexual intercourse of 122 ± 7.1 beats/minute and 124 ± 7.2 during other activities.[12]

One group[13] compared the cardiovascular response to sexual intercourse with stair climbing. For this, nine men without and eight men with coronary artery disease (average age fifty years) were studied. The stair test involved walking for 10 minutes then climbing twenty-two stairs in 10 seconds (the average English flight is twelve to thirteen). In normal subjects the mean maximal heart rate was 123 ± 8 beats/minutes during intercourse and 122 ± 5 beats/minute on the stairs, while in the coronary patients it was 118 ± 6 and 115 ± 7 beats/minute, respectively. The systo-

131

lic blood pressure rose modestly to 146 ± 2 mmHg in the normal subjects for both stresses but in the coronary patients it was actually less during intercourse (144 ± 6 mmHg) than on the stairs (164 ± 7 mmHg; $p < 0.01$).

A pattern of cardiovascular responses emerges. For the long married or cohabiting couple (one assumes this can be so for homosexual as well as heterosexual relationships), the heart rate and blood pressure response is modest, achieving its maximum at orgasm. For middle-aged couples this occurs on average twice a week, with the maximal response representing only 15 seconds or so of the 16 minutes' average duration of sexual intercourse—representing less than 0.3 per cent of leisure time.[10]

It must be remembered that the cardiovascular response to sexual intercourse will be more vigorous (and more frequent) in the younger age group, which may present problems with an age mismatch (eg, old man, young bride). It will be exaggerated in an unfamiliar environment with a casual partner and will increase following any rise in baseline levels of cardiac demand, for example, after a large meal or hot bath.

It is important though to establish that sexual intercourse is part of the normal lifestyle of an individual, whether he or she has coronary disease or not. As in any form of exercise, myocardial demand (heart rate and blood pressure) will increase. With appropriate background information the physician or nurse can place the demand in context, reassure the needlessly concerned and by simple tests (eg, climbing two flights of stairs) enable individuals to lead full and satisfactory lives.

Work

Up to 90 per cent of people can return to their previous occupation. Specific advice will be needed for heavy goods vehicle and public service vehicle licence holders and those doing heavy manual work. Heavy goods vehicle and public service vehicle licence holders must surrender their licences (it is their responsibility, not the doctor's) but after a period of time, providing exercise ECGs and angiography are satisfactory, a licence may be restored. A panel of cardiologists assess the

Table 13.2 Coronary home exercise programmes to be followed during week after discharge

Name: _____

	Day 1	Day 2	Day 3	Day 4	Day 5	Day 6	Day 7
Leg: straight lift lying down							
Arms: raise and lower sideways							
Knee: bend and straighten lying down							
Side bending while standing							
Squat for lifting practice							

Go for a short walk each day, gradually increasing the distance and keep up a fairly brisk pace.
For the first few days use the stairs only at night and in the morning then gradually increase their use during the day.
Always rest if you feel any chest pain or faint, or are short of breath
Tick each box as programme completed.

cases on individual merit. The disablement resettlement office may be able to help where possible and, providing finances are available in the current employment situation, early retirement may be the most sensible option. It must be made clear to the patient that this does not mean we are concerned about him medically.

Travel

About four to six weeks after an infarct most patients are fit to drive and certainly if they have had a satisfactory treadmill exercise ECG. They should inform the driving licence authorities of their infarct and check the conditions of their car insurance policies. They should avoid the stress of rush hour traffic

Table 13.3 Rehabilitation programme Coronary outpatients

Name: _____ Age: _____ Date of coronary: _____
Date: _____

Pulse rate: Before exercise After After a 5-minute rest															
1 **Standing** Trunk side bending															
2 **Standing** Trunk rotation															
3 **Standing** Alternate knees to chest															
4 **Standing** Arms circling with 1.8 kg (4 lbs)															
5 **Lying** Straight lift alternate legs															
6 **Prone lying** Straight lift alternate legs															
7 **Lying with knees bent up** Raise bottom															
8 **Lying** Lift medicine ball from chest															
9 **Lying** Head & shoulders lift sitting															
10 **Squats**															
11 **Step-ups**															
12 **Cycle**															

Tick box as exercises completed.

133

initially. Air travel is safe from six weeks but may be undertaken earlier if essential, preferably after seeking expert advice.

HEART FAILURE

This is one of the more difficult aspects of rehabilitation. If the failure reflects valvar damage and medical therapy is unsuccessful, valve replacement can be dramatically beneficial. When the problem is heart muscle disease from whatever cause, controlling symptoms at the same time as maintaining activity requires the early use of vasodilator drugs.[14]

Conventional therapy of heart failure involves diuretics and, in appropriate cases, digoxin. Diuretics are excellent in reducing volume and relieving breathlessness and certainly in mild heart failure this will be all that is necessary. However, as the need for diuretics increases so the volume decreases until the critical balance between blood returning to the heart and blood leaving it is reduced too far. Breathlessness will be resolved but cardiac output will not be increased and the dry-skinned, dehydrated, tired and lethargic individual will result.

By using vasodilator drugs early, the blood returning to the heart (preload) can be reduced and the blood leaving the heart have the resistance reduced (afterload) thereby facilitating cardiac output. A 25–30 per cent improvement in performance can be achieved without the social inconvenience and debility of excessive diuresis. This therapy is available in hospital practice and the quality of life benefits are exceptional for a substantial number.

Patients languishing on high dose diuretics need a re-evaluation; they should be sought out.

CARDIAC SURGERY

The immediate problem is musculoskeletal pain from the thoracic spine and anterior chest wall. The patients need to be aware that this is going to happen and again booklets supplement the advice given by doctors and nursing staff. The pain resolves slowly but in a small but significant number persists and interferes with mobilization. Here a two- to four-week course of non-steroidal anti-inflammatory agents is very helpful.

Surgical patients are in hospital an average of ten days and on discharge are mobile, climbing stairs, and so forth. It is important to emphasize to the patient and spouse that they have not had an illness but had one prevented or corrected. They cannot undo the good of the operation—it will not fall apart. Sexual relations can be resumed as desired but the sternal pain may be limiting. The side-to-side position or mutual masturbation will usually circumvent these problems. A small pillow placed between chests can greatly reduce the discomfort, not only from the sternal scar but from the discomfort felt by the woman as her partner's chest hairs regrow.

Returning to driving, walking, swimming is again as early as possible with the emphasis most positively on resuming normal life, with a return to work at approximately twelve weeks. Patients should be warned about occasional muscle pains, particularly with front wheel drive cars which do not have power-assisted steering. I frequently use the myocardial infarct rehabilitation programme if progress at six weeks is not as quick as it should be. The reason is invariably lack of confidence and enrolment in a rehabilitation programme is a great confidence booster.

WOMEN'S PROBLEMS

This is not a sexist section. Women still do the housework; they feel houseproud. If they have a heart attack the husband and the family must rally round to help relieve the patient of these commitments in the early

134

stages. After heart surgery, during sexual intercourse with the woman underneath there can be enormous fears of inducing damage, or giving rise to pain—these fears must be allayed and the pain treated. A fact of life is the increased incidence of heart disease in men, still the breadwinner in most homes. The spouse may need help to manage while the partner is in hospital (here relatives can come to stay or the older children be encouraged to contribute). A good family doctor is most invaluable for simply listening, as is a good neighbour.

Cardiac illness is a family problem. All members need open simple advice about what is happening, what will be happening and how everyone including the patient can contribute. Even without access to a formal rehabilitation programme most people will manage with education and commonsense. It is the medical profession's responsibility to provide this basis for recovery.

PRACTICAL POINTS

- Rehabilitation begins with the onset of symptoms.

- Talking to patients and relatives *frequently* is an essential part of management.

- Advice should be routinely given but is often misunderstood in the stressful atmosphere. Booklets are a repetitive source of information and should be used automatically.

- Sexual activity is equivalent to briskly going up and down two flights of household stairs.

- Work is usually returned to two months postinfarction.

- Inarticulate people, those with limited intelligence and racial groups with a poor command of English need more patience and more tolerance.

14
Myocardial infarction—secondary prevention

BACKGROUND

Secondary prevention is concerned with reducing morbidity and mortality in patients who have already been documented to have coronary artery disease (CAD). Those who have one event (angina, infarction or arrhythmia) are more likely than the general population to experience another. In the same way as we manage the angina patient we need to establish who is at risk (prognosis) and whether the risk can be modified or abolished (intervention).

EVALUATION

Prognosis

Most patients who survive the first hours and days after infarction pursue an uncomplicated course. Taken overall, those with anterior infarction do less well than those with inferior infarction because of a greater muscle loss. The hospital mortality is related to haemodynamic status on arrival. Those with a normal blood pressure and no evidence of heart failure have a low hospital mortality, usually less than 10 per cent. Death here usually follows an arrhythmia, infarct extension in the recovery period or a sudden mechanical complication such as rupture of the myocardium, ventricular septum or papillary muscle. Those with cardiogenic shock have a near hopeless course with a mortality close to 100 per cent. Those with left ventricular failure but a normal or raised blood pressure have a mortality of up to 30 per cent.

Longterm mortality has been the subject of detailed study. The overall one-year morta-lity is 10–15 per cent; however, up to 50 per cent of these deaths occur in the first three months.[1] In one study, one-third of deaths occurred in the first six weeks.[2] Early evaluation is needed if events are to be modified.

The coronary prognostic index of Norris[3] has related survival to age at infarct, presence or absence of cardiac enlargement or pulmonary congestion on the first chest x-ray examination and presence or absence of a previous infarct. This has held true for follow-up to three, six and, in the latest report, fifteen years[4] (see Figures 14.1–14.5). Nothing can be done about age but the size of infarct may be reducible by intervention with thrombolysis (see page 126).

INFARCT SIZE   The size of the infarct dictates prognosis. In the study by Norris et al., patients with a good prognostic index had a 36 per cent mortality rate at fifteen years and those with a poor index 70 per cent. This observation has been supported by many other studies and an ejection fraction of less than 50 per cent and certainly less than 40 per cent has an adverse prognosis.[5] Given that about 50 per cent of infarct survivors have an ejection fraction less than 50 per cent, there is obviously a large pool of patients able to be identified as being at risk. In addition, 80 per cent of these have coronary arteries suitable for bypass surgery and benefit from operation is possible.[5] About 10 per cent of patients will have clinically evident cardiac failure, but 10 per cent may have similar reduced left ventricular function which is not clinically obvious. If the peak CPK-MB is greater than three times the normal limit this is evidence of significant muscle loss though of course a smaller rise on the background of a previous infarct may reflect significant additive muscle loss. Further evaluation of these patients by echo-cardiography or radionuclide ventriculography may show a reduced ejection fraction, indicating an adverse prognosis in the first year (>25 per cent mortality)[6] (see Table 14.1).

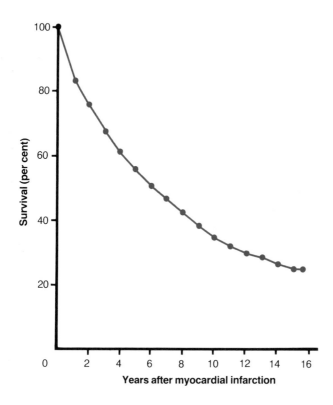

Figure 14.1 Survival of 530 patients after recovery from myocardial infarction.

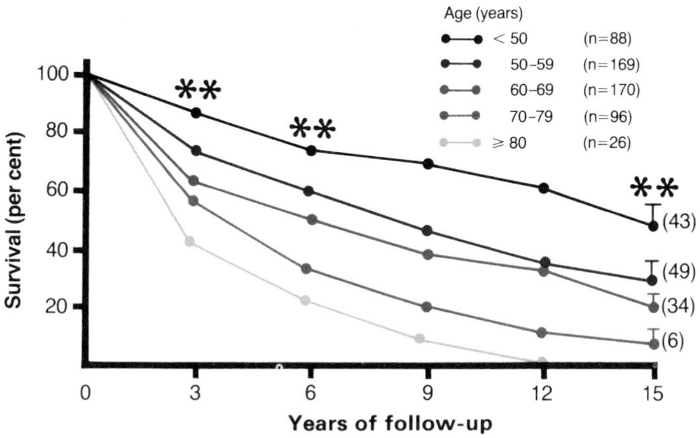

Figure 14.2 Survival related to age at time of infarction. ** = Significant difference.

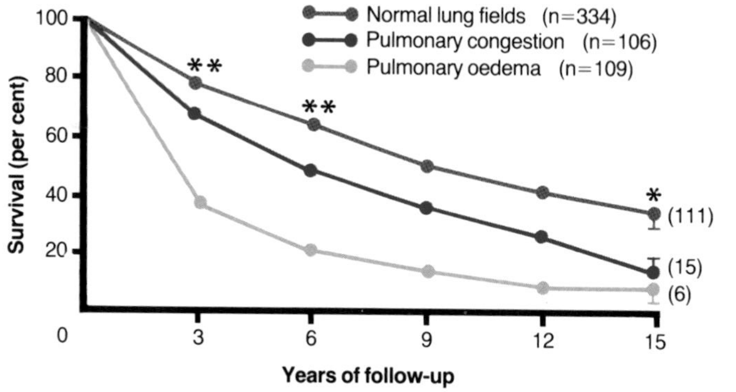

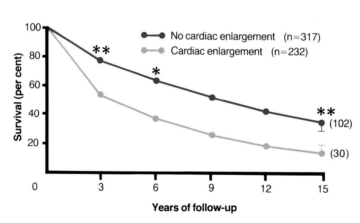

Figure 14.3 Survival related to pulmonary congestion on chest x-ray.

Figure 14.4 Survival related to cardiomegaly on chest x-ray.

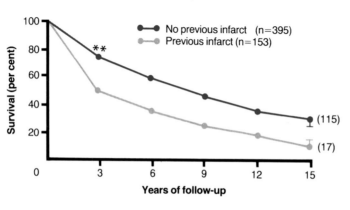

Figure 14.5 Survival related to previous infarction.

∗ or ∗∗ = Significant differences.

ANGINA Angina after infarction has a high mortality rate. The risk factor is easily identifiable by what the patient is telling you. For the patient angina means heart disease and the mortality rate at three months can be as high as 25 per cent. In one study at six months it was 57 per cent in the absence of a reduced ejection fraction.[8] Medical treatment and early angiography is indicated for these patients who represent 10 per cent of the population of infarct survivors. Though they may stabilize on medical therapy, high risk anatomy needs exclusion in case prognostic surgery (or possibly angioplasty) is necessary.

ISCHAEMIA AND A GOOD VENTRICLE Patients with an uncomplicated infarct have a favourable one-year mortality of less than 10 per cent. Within this group, however, is a high risk subset who on early exercise testing show significant ST segment depression in leads other than those involved in the infarct. On average those with a normal postinfarct exercise ECG have a one-year mortality of less than 3 per cent, while those who have a positive exercise ECG have a one-year mortality of about 20 per cent.[9–11] The exercise variables of ST depression greater than 1 mm angina at a low workload and a significant fall

in systolic blood pressure and/or rise in diastolic blood pressure identify jeopardized myocardium and the need for angiography to document the anatomy. Because of early deaths, the earlier the stress test the better and this should be carried out routinely on all uncomplicated infarcts within three weeks of infarction.

In our studies of the value of early exercise testing in identifying the presence or absence of significant additional CAD to that which subtended the infarct, we achieved an accuracy greater than 90 per cent in both, stating with an abnormal test that there was disease and with a normal test that there was not additional disease. We therefore related the ST segment change to the anatomy as well as the prognosis.[12] It is estimated that 30 per cent of all patients surviving infarcts are at risk from additional ischaemia. In our studies of *uncomplicated* infarcts with no significant left ventricular damage the incidence was 45 per cent.[13] We intervened with bypass surgery and recorded a mortality at three years of 2 per cent against the predicted one-year mortality of 20 per cent.[13] Our results are based on early maximal exercise testing using a twelve-lead ECG in the absence of drugs such as beta-blockers which might affect the ST segment.

Table 14.1 The fate of 100 typical postinfarct survivors at Day 14

Number of patients	Annual mortality per cent	Reason
50	2	Good left ventricular function, normal exercise ECG
30	10–25	Rest or exercise ischaemia but good left ventricular function
20	> 25	Heart failure, or CPK > 500 units/litre and/or ejection fraction < 40 per cent

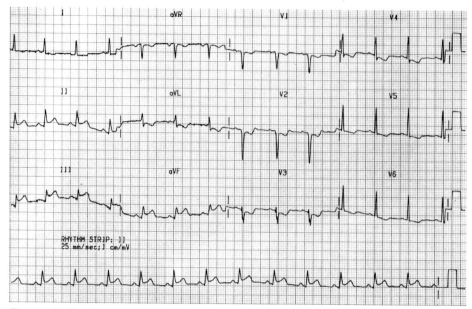

Figure 14.6 Acute inferior infarction with anterior reciprocal ST depression.

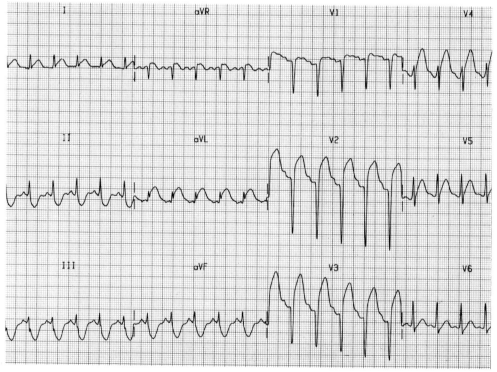

Figure 14.7 Anterior infarction with inferior reciprocal ST depression.

We have also evaluated the use of 'reciprocal' ST segment depression at the time of infarction using one of three ECGs recorded in the first 24 hours.[14] The presence of reciprocal ST change had previously been shown to be associated with a high risk of fatal arrhythmia and late morbidity[15] but we took this a step further to correlate it with the exercise ECG and angiogram. Reciprocal ST depression is depression of 1 mm or more in the ECG leads other than those reflecting the infarct (see Figures 14.6 and 14.7). Reciprocal ST depression could at a very early stage identify patients with severe coronary disease, and when it did a significant number (70 per cent) became symptomatic subsequently, with over 50 per cent needing bypass surgery. In contrast, of those without reciprocal change only 15 per cent became symptomatic with 7 per cent needing surgery. However, the reciprocal ST segment change did fail to identify some patients with multivessel disease who were subsequently detected by exercise testing. Thus, in the clinical context for hospitals with limited facilities, reciprocal ST depression should be considered a marker of severe multivessel coronary arterial disease and a risk factor for subsequent cardiac events. When no reciprocal change is present early exercise testing provides valuable additional information and should be done routinely. Coronary arteriography should follow where indicated.

ARRHYTHMIAS Ambulatory ECGs are used to record ventricular arrhythmias and are more accurate and practical than conventional bedside monitoring. The presence of complex ventricular arrhythmias is more frequent with extensive infarction.[16] Complex arrhythmias are associated with a 15 per cent one-year mortality in contrast with only 5 per cent for those with simple ventricular extrasystoles.[17] However, this survival difference only occurs when heart failure is present (ie, left ventricular dysfunction) and complex arrhythmias

alone are not a strong predictor of events.[17] In other words complex ventricular arrhythmias are a marker of left ventricular dysfunction and it is the latter that determines the prognosis. While antiarrhythmics in these high risk groups fail to influence mortality (see page 186), there is no doubt that symptomatic arrhythmias should be recorded and treated, if not to improve the quantity then the quality of life.

The flow diagram on page 142 modified from Epstein et al.[18] provides a practical evaluation plan regarding secondary prevention.

TREATMENT

The major problem in assessing intervention studies is the absence of objective baseline data to indicate risk. None are stratified on positive or negative postinfarct exercise tests. From these studies it is known that after infarction 50 per cent of patients will do well without intervention. By taking a diffuse postinfarct population we have either under- or overvalued the intervention because of dilution with people who are not at risk. Thus we know that beta-blockers are beneficial but surely not in those with only a one-year risk of less than 3 per cent. It is important therefore when looking at invervention data to place them in the context of the already established high and low risk groups and not to blanket manage the postinfarct patient. Given the 15–25 per cent reduction in mortality at one year as a result of beta-blockade postinfarction, it should be asked of other agents what do they have to add, rather than whether they can provide an alternative.

Risk factors

The risk factors for primary prevention apply to secondary prevention but the responses may be different.

Cigarette smoking

To stop smoking is the single most important

contribution the patient can make to his own future. The mortality is reduced by 50 per cent at five years.[19,20] It has been estimated that 28 per cent of deaths among male smokers who continue to smoke after infarction can be directly related to the cigarettes.[21] Passive smoking may well be perilous[22] and all efforts should be made to reduce cigarette smoke in the environment.

Diet

Although losing weight may make the patient feel better and perhaps help if angina is a problem, unfortunately there is no evidence that weight reduction or cholesterol modification influences mortality. Several trials of diet and/or lipid-lowering agents have been undertaken and a detailed review of their results has provided no evidence of prolongation of life postinfarct.[23] Attention has been drawn to the adverse effects of drug therapy (see page 25).

It would seem sensible to adopt a prudent enjoyable diet and try to achieve optimum weight for height. None of the trials has addressed the problem of the patients with familial hypercholesterolaemia, who have only been studied on a primary prevention basis (see page 24). Strict dietary policies should be advocated here and the use of the patient to identify family members who may be at risk.

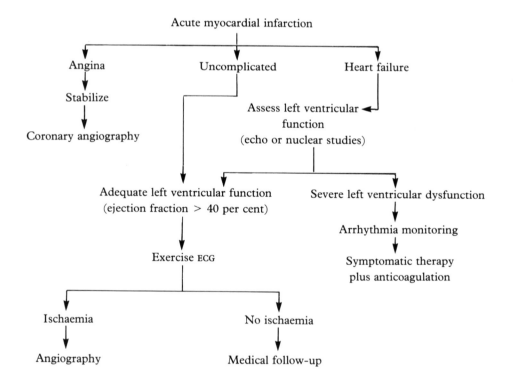

NB. In the absence of readily available exercise testing, significant reciprocal ST depression greater than 2 mm indicates the need for early angiography.

Hypertension

There is no clear evidence that hypertensive therapy will benefit subsequent cardiac events after infarction, but as the control of hypertension is sensible with regard to reducing strokes and possibly angina and heart failure, treatment remains logical.

Physical exercise

Six prospective studies exist concerning the effects of physical exercise training after myocardial infarction.[23] The exercise programmes formed a component of an attempt at lifestyle change which included diet and smoking. Five of the studies indicated a possible preventive benefit (up to 20 per cent reduction in mortality) but numbers overall were small and compliance poor. Thus, if the patient wishes to get fit he should be encouraged to do so. If he hates exercise there is no mandate to make him suffer it. It is no use jogging if it is hated; better to walk in the countryside, swim, dance, or play tennis. Some prefer golf; others would sooner sit and fish. There has to be enjoyment or stress will be all that is achieved.

Personality

There is no relationship between type A behaviour and longterm outcome of acute myocardial infarction during follow up for one to three years.[24] Stress supplements other risk factors rather than acting as a powerful risk factor on its own. Certainly severe stress can cause a cardiac event providing there is an underlying problem.[2] Those under stress are recommended to try to make certain lifestyle changes to reduce stress (see Chapter 13). Booklets are available to help the patient and relatives, and can supplement the advice given at consultation. Stress reduction must therefore be part of a commonsense approach to life rather than a scientific belief in benefit.

Beta-blockade

The trials of timolol and propranolol,[26] which reported a reduction in mortality at one year of the order of 25 per cent, lead to the recommendation that beta-blockade should be considered for all survivors of myocardial infarction. This is considered to be inappropriate for those with a risk of less than 3 per cent at one year. The recommendation reflects the lack of objective baseline entry data for residual ischaemia and risk.

Here we are concerned with late intervention, ie, the start of oral beta-blockade two to three days after the infarct. Immediate intravenous beta-blockade has been discussed previously (see page 104). A review of thirteen published trials has identified a mortality benefit of between 15 and 25 per cent.[27] Given a placebo risk of, say, eight patients a year beta-blockade will only help a further two. However, in the higher risk subset with abnormal exercise ECGs expecting a 20 per cent mortality, beta-blockade may help a further five. Knowing the adverse effects of beta-blockade we can thus be more selective in our use in order to confer the greatest benefit. Furthermore, we must realize that only a half of infarct survivors will be suitable for beta-blockade because of contraindications.

The flow diagram in Figure 14.8 reflects my use of beta-blockade after the infarct. All suitable cases should start oral therapy but only until more objective assessments are made. Beta-blockers give time to manage patients properly as well as being definitive in a small subgroup.

Which one should be used? Convincing evidence exists for propranolol 80 mg bd[26] and timolol 10 mg bd.[25] The study of sotalol 320 mg once a day was less positive.[28] It is interesting that beta-blockers with intrinsic sympathomimetic activity (ISA) show no benefit (oxprenolol[29] and pindolol[30]) in late studies. I favour a simple regime and use atenolol 50 mg daily. I do not identify benefit between drugs (all comparisons are versus pacebo) but it seems wise to avoid drugs with ISA and adopt a simple regime (once- or twice-daily).

143

Benefit may be due to an antiarrhythmic action since sudden death is reduced by 30 per cent and in the propranolol study 24-hour ECGs showed less complex ventricular arrhythmias. This, however, may reflect the varying degrees of left ventricular dysfunction at entry—there is no stratification based on this. In experimental studies beta-blockers raise the threshold to ventricular fibrillation.[31] Furthermore, a more severe and rapid metabolic disorder has been shown experimentally in dogs to lead to ventricular fibrillation after coronary artery ligation.[32] That is, the rate of developing ischaemia rather than the amount may relate to sudden death and an agent which influences this rate favourably may

therefore affect prognosis. This has been shown previously for beta-blockers in patients with angina and it is feasible that on occasions the ischaemic state may be reached so fast that the pain level is bypassed quickly and ventricular fibrillation occurs (see Figure 14.9).[33] I have so far advocated the use of beta-blockade, but the next question is for how long. Clearly those who are at low risk can be stopped after the exercise test.[34] Those with residual ischaemia who are not severe enough or suitable for surgery should be treated indefinitely and doses adjusted if symptoms develop. Benefit has been recorded for six years with timolol[35] and three years with metoprolol.[36] They should be continued

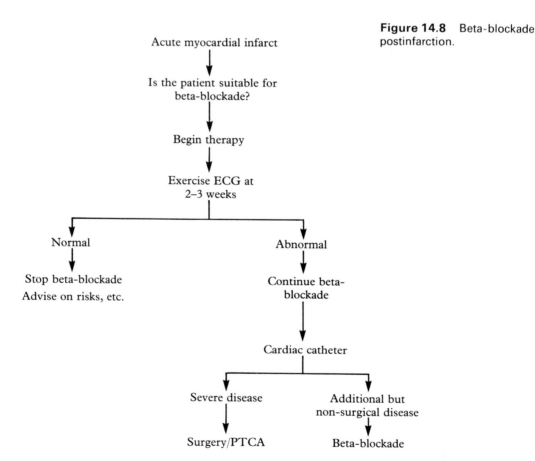

Figure 14.8 Beta-blockade postinfarction.

Acute myocardial infarct

Is the patient suitable for beta-blockade?

Begin therapy

Exercise ECG at 2–3 weeks

Normal

Stop beta-blockade
Advise on risks, etc.

Abnormal

Continue beta-blockade

Cardiac catheter

Severe disease

Surgery/PTCA

Additional but non-surgical disease

Beta-blockade

in those awaiting surgery until the operation is carried out.

Antiarrhythmics

These have been discussed already but will be repeated for completeness; there is no evidence that antiarrhythmic agents other than beta-blockers confer any advantage on mortality in spite of evidence that they reduce ventricular arrhythmias recorded on 24-hour ECGs.[23]

Anticoagulants

No convincing trials have been published to justify longterm anticoagulation routinely postinfarction.[23,37] No trial has been capable of detecting even a 20 per cent reduction in mortality. One of the most recent, the Dutch Sixty-Plus Reinfarction Trial, was concerned with the effects of stopping therapy rather than initiating it.[38] By removing withdrawals and protocol deviants a benefit was seen for those continuing anticoagulants, though side-effects were not infrequent. It can be concluded that a patient who has been on warfarin for years postinfarction without side-effects should continue—but little else. Of course anticoagulants should be used for those with specific indications, eg, embolization. When comparing anticoagulants with aspirin there was no difference in mortality or non-fatal infarct,[39] but unfortunately no placebo group was included.

Antiplatelet agents

Sulphinpyrazone was initially believed to be effective but major trial defects were

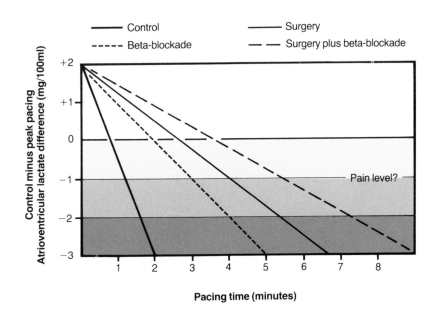

Figure 14.9 The rate of development of myocardial ischaemia may be modified by the therapeutic manoeuvres. It may be that the faster the ischaemia develops the more vulnerable the patient is to ventricular fibrillation. Depending on individual pain levels, ischaemia may be silent for varying degrees of time.

discovered and a subsequent study was inconclusive.[40,41]

Dipyridamole and aspirin were evaluated jointly in the Persantin Aspirin Reinfarction Study (PARIS)[42] and aspirin alone in the Aspirin Myocardial Infarction Study (AMIS).[43] No reduction in mortality was seen for either. Thus there is no evidence at present to support the routine use of antiplatelet therapy postinfarction, though further studies of varying doses of aspirin are under way.

Calcium antagonists

Verapamil has been studied in Denmark[44] in patients postinfarction and compared with placebo. It was administered intravenously then orally 120 mg tid. There was no difference in the incidence of reinfarction or mortality at six and twelve months.

A trial of nifedipine 10 mg qds versus placebo[45] was undertaken in 4488 patients. There was an overall increase in mortality of 8 per cent in the nifedipine group though confidence intervals varied from $+30$ per cent to -14 per cent. Subgroup analysis identified no benefit.

Calcium antagonists cannot be recommended routinely postinfarction as monotherapy. It is not known if nifedipine plus beta-blockade, ie, combination therapy, will be more effective than beta-blockade alone. Results with diltiazem are still awaited.

PRACTICAL POINTS

- The secondary prevention of myocardial infarction relies on an understanding of the factors that influence prognosis—extent of left ventricular damage and residual ischaemia.

- Patients can be stratified into high and low risk on clinical grounds and by postinfarction exercise testing.

- Angiography and surgery have an important role to play in reducing morbidity and mortality.

- The only drugs of proven benefit are beta-blockers.

- Low risk patients need no specific therapy other than advice on lifestyle, especially stopping smoking.

15
Subendocardial infarction

A separate chapter has been allocated for subendocardial (non-Q-wave) infarction because there is a dangerous complacency about its management. This reflects the belief that the infarct must be smaller because it is not transmural (full thickness) and the knowledge that the short-term survival rate is better.[1] The main concern is that the incidence of further infarction, both early and late, and sudden death is higher after subendocardial infarction, indicating a high risk group.[2] Comparing transmural with subendocardial infarction at four-year follow-up, 12 per cent of patients with anterior transmural, 22 per cent with inferior transmural and 57 per cent with subendocardial infarcts had recurrent infarcts.[1] In the subendocardial group, in most instances the second event was at the site of the first, supporting the idea that subendocardial infarction was an intermediate stage between unstable angina and transmural infarction.[2]

Clinically subendocardial infarction is defined on the basis of the ECG. It is a myocardial infarction not involving the QRS complex (non-Q-wave infarction) but usually resulting in deep symmetrically depressed T waves (see Figure 15.1).[3] This is not pathologically precise, however, because it can be found frequently in the elderly at post-mortem examination[4] without ECG changes, and although the T wave change is found in 88 per cent of subendocardial infarcts it also occurs in 40 per cent of transmural infarcts.[5] However, it remains a working clinical definition associated at one year with a 21 per cent incidence of progression to full thickness infarction.[2]

The most worrying group are those in whom a subendocardial infarct follows previous myocardial damage. Here the size of the infarct cannot be predicted from the ECG because the old Q waves may mask any new ones. Again the outcome will be dependent on the amount of left ventricular damage. In one study those with first-time subendocardial infarcts had no hospital or first-year mortality, while those with pre-existing disease had an in-hospital mortality of 13 per cent and a further 22 per cent died within one year.[1]

AETIOLOGY

This concerns the patient who presents with myocardial infarction in the usual way and in whom the aetiology is invariably coronary atheroma. Other causes of subendocardial infarction include aortic valve disease, pulmonary embolism and subarachnoid haemorrhage.[6] It has also been recorded after prolonged resuscitation[7] when the coronary arteries were normal and it represents half of the post-operative (general surgery) infarcts occurring in those with and without pre-existing disease.[8] Here the sequence most likely reflects an imbalance between coronary perfusion (aortic valve disease, resuscitation) and noradrenaline-induced increased demand (subarachnoid haemorrhage, operation).

As most deaths and subsequent infarcts occur late[1] these are therefore amenable to modification. Given that the subendocardial incidence is 20–30 per cent of the total infarct population, there is a substantial subgroup in whom there is an opportunity to modify prognosis.[9] In contrast with fatal transmural

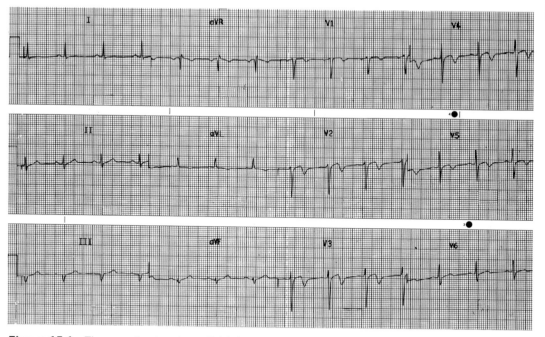

Figure 15.1   The ECG of subendocardial infarction. T-wave inversion is seen in leads V1–V5.

infarcts where total occlusion of the coronary artery occurred in 95 per cent, in subendocardial infarcts 87 per cent were patent.[10] The pathophysiology suggests a mixture of thrombosis, partial occlusion, and total occlusion but damage limited by collaterals and vasoconstriction. In most instances, partial occlusion must be operative from the patency figures.[10] This means that while deaths remain likely to reflect ventricular fibrillation, those who survive are likely to have patent arteries beyond a stenotic lesion, rendering surgery possible.

MANAGEMENT

My management strategy reflects the belief that a surgical (or perhaps angioplasty) option may improve prognosis. Patients are stabilized in the usual way for myocardial infarc-

tion and before discharge from hospital angiography is carried out to document the anatomy in all suitable patients up to sixty-five years of age. They are treated with aspirin as for unstable angina although it is accepted that there is no scientific support for this, but the mechanism is similar. Because a lot of evidence points to thrombosis, many recommend heparin for 24 hours and trials of thrombolytic therapy are being proposed.[11] Beta-blockade or calcium antagonists and nitrate therapy should be started routinely. In a multicentre double-blind randomized trial of diltiazem 90 mg 6 hourly (287 patients) there was a significant reduction in reinfarction at 14 days but no difference in mortality compared with placebo (289 patients).[12] Eighty per cent of the patients were coprescribed nitrates and 60 per cent beta-blockers. Whilst adverse effects were few, eight diltiazem

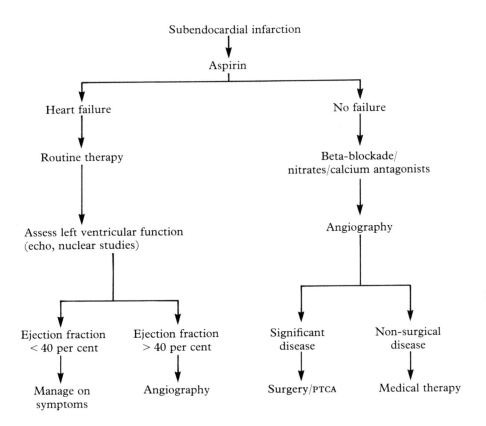

Figure 15.2 Management strategy.

patients had second degree heart block, of whom six were receiving beta-blockade. This contrasts with two in the placebo group, one of whom was taking beta-blockers. There was a reassuring absence of significant left ventricular dysfunction in the diltiazem group even when combined with beta-blockade. Since treatment is hospital-based with cardiac care unit monitoring, until further data on other calcium antagonists are available diltiazem

should be used in all suitable cases with non-Q-wave infarction.

After stabilization, or sooner if pain continues, all patients of appropriate age and physical health should undergo angiography. If anatomically they are surgical or angioplasty candidates they should be referred for early operation, maintaining medical therapy even if they have no symptoms. Based on the data concerning prognosis, this aggressive op-

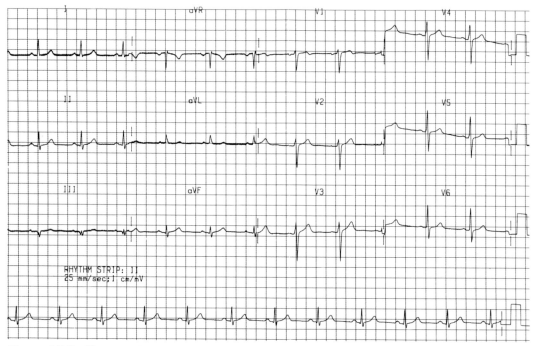

Figure 15.3   The ECG of patient in Figure 15.1 showing normal T waves at six months. This emphasizes the importance of always looking at an ECG sequence, not an isolated reading.

tion seems sensible until controlled trials are undertaken to validate other options. This strategy is summarized in Figure 15.2. On follow-up, the ECGs may well revert to normal (see Figure 15.3), which should not lull the doctors into a false sense of security but should emphasize the importance of reviewing an ECG sequence rather than an isolated recording.

PRACTICAL POINTS

- The assumption of smaller infarction being safe is wrong.

- Subendocardial infarction frequently progresses to full thickness infarction.

- Aspirin and heparin may be of benefit but are not proven.

- After medical stabilization more detailed assessment is needed before discharge (see Figure 15.2).

16
Silent ischaemia

BACKGROUND

Silent ischaemia is defined as objective evidence of ischaemia (eg, ST depression) without pain or other recognized complaints. It can occur in people who are never symptomatic when it may be detected by chance on ambulatory monitoring, treadmill exercise testing or routine twelve-lead ECG (silent infarction). It may also present for the first time as sudden death. In those who have symptoms, silent ischaemia can also occur in the presence of stable and unstable angina as well as after a classic myocardial infarction.

SIGNIFICANCE

Intermittent asymptomatic ST depression is well recognized[1] but believed to be unusual in the normal population.[2] In the coronary population the presence of silent ischaemic episodes (see Figure 16.1) is the subject of many investigative studies to establish its significance. Early reports established the accuracy of ambulatory ECG monitoring in detecting ST depression, correlating the findings with angiographically proven coronary artery disease (CAD).[3,4] More recently the frequency, severity and duration of silent ischaemic episodes has been shown to reflect more severe CAD, ie, the more disease there is the more silent ischaemia is seen.[5]

The rationale for treating silent ischaemia *per se* must come from evidence that silent ischaemia alone has adverse prognostic implications. Only in unstable angina does this appear to be true at present. In one study, greater than 60 minutes of silent ischaemia in 24 hours identified a group with a 60 per cent chance of a further cardiac event within one month of presenting.[6]

Of interest, the distribution of coronary lesions was similar in those with and without silent ischaemia, raising the possibility that in this situation silent ischaemia was acting as a marker of continuing vasomotor instability and thus the need for more active intervention.

In patients with stable angina 75 per cent of episodes of ST depression are painless.[7] There is no specific prognostic information available concerning silent ischaemia in this group, whose prognosis has already been evaluated by treadmill exercise testing. It seems unlikely that monitoring for silent ischaemia will provide any advantage above and beyond exercise testing, which is a cheaper, shorter and less labour-intensive means of risk evaluation.

It is not known why pain will occur on some occasions and not on others. Perhaps it is not the amount of ischaemia but the speed with which it develops (see page 145).

MANAGEMENT

Antianginal medication and bypass surgery reduce the episodes of both silent and painful ischaemia.[8,9] We need to know if it matters when a patient is feeling well on therapy but has residual silent ischaemia. In the presence of unstable angina I have already advocated an angiographic approach (page 73) but when there is doubt concerning the functional significance of the lesions ambulatory monitoring may provide useful additional information concerning the extent of ischaemia, and influence management and prognosis. Most patients, however, either have stable angina or are free of symptoms.

In stable patients silent episodes of ST depression of 2 mm or greater, a total period of over 60 minutes in 48 hours and more than 6 episodes in 48 hours are believed to reflect high risk.[10] However we have no evidence that this is a superior prognostic marker to the treadmill exercise ECG.

Beta-blockade has been shown to reduce mortality at one year in postmyocardial infarction patients and risk can also be related to the early postinfarct exercise ECG. It is conceivable that beta-blockade may be anti-ischaemic and reduce silent and painful ischaemic episodes but there is no evidence to support this case. Furthermore, it is difficult to believe that mortality can be further reduced by addressing our energies to any residual silent ischaemic episodes. However in the first two to three weeks after infarction before the routine treadmill ECG, there may be a role for ambulatory monitoring of the ST segment to see whether it identifies an at-risk group who need early angiography. There is clearly a need for such a study.

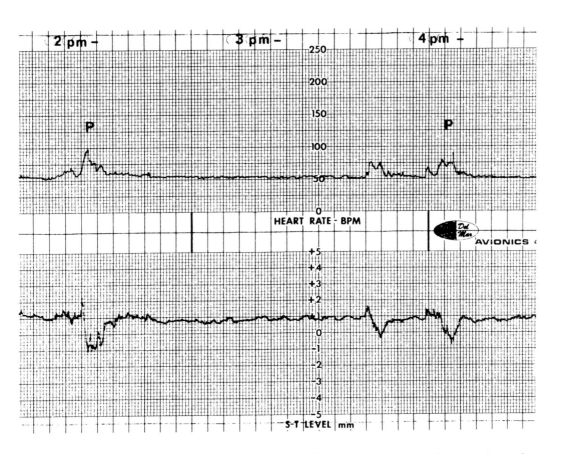

Figure 16.1 Trend plot of heart rate (top) and ST level from ambulatory recordings. ST depression occurs on two occasions with pain (P) but not on the other.

At present it is simply not known whether asymptomatic ST depression should be identified and abolished. I suspect there may be a role in the more acute settings but only en route to more definitive investigations and action. In addition it may be helpful to perform ambulatory ST monitoring for patients who cannot exercise readily, and for those who have atypical chest pains and an equivocal exercise ECG. It clearly can be of great value when Prinzmetal's angina is suspected, when nocturnal ST elevation may be silent or painful.

At present there is no evidence to suggest that for the majority of ischaemic patients our management needs modification as a result of the detection of silent ischaemia. Nor do we have a mandate to perform routine and expensive screening to identify it. It is not, however, to be dismissed.

PRACTICAL POINTS

- Silent ischaemia is common.

- It appears to identify an adverse prognosis in unstable angina.

- In stable patients its significance is unknown.

- Early postinfarction it has not been evaluated.

- Ambulatory ST monitoring may be of value in selected patients (eg, poor mobility, nocturnal pain).

- There is no evidence at present that routine and expensive screening is worthwhile.

17
Chronic heart failure

BACKGROUND

The management of acute left heart failure is discussed in Chapter 12 (see page 106). This chapter is concerned with chronic cardiac failure caused by substantial heart muscle damage.

Heart failure can be defined as the pathophysiological state which arises when cardiac function fails to meet peripheral demands, ie, the supply of blood leaving the heart (cardiac output) is insufficient to meet the body's metabolic demands from normal activity. The development of cardiac failure, with or without ischaemia as the cause, is associated with a poor prognosis. When substantial heart muscle damage occurs it may be secondary to a large infarction or reflect chronic ischaemia. This latter state usually results in a poorly functioning ventricle with a globar reduction in function rather like a congestive cardiomyopathy. The cause is fibrosis secondary to coronary arterial disease (CAD), also known as ischaemic cardiomyopathy.[1] In the absence of diabetes it is not known why coronary disease presents as heart failure in some and as angina or infarction in others. Unfortunately, however, the heart failure state is associated with a poor prognosis. In one study[2] the mortality at one year was 31 per cent and at five years 84 per cent. Similar figures arose from the Framingham study, with a 50 per cent five-year survival and 10 per cent ten-year survival.[3]

In spite of the many available therapeutic options, until the beginning of 1986 no studies existed which showed any benefits on prognosis. Emphasis has always been on improving well-being. This changed with the publication of the Veterans Administrative Co-operative Study.[4] This study was designed to evaluate the effects of vasodilator therapy on mortality among patients with moderate congestive cardiac failure who were already receiving digoxin and diuretics. The therapeutic regimes are unusual but the results of importance. Six hundred and forty-two men were randomized to receive placebo, prazosin 20 mg daily or the combination of isosorbide dinitrate (160 mg daily) and hydralazine (300 mg daily). After two years the hydralazine/nitrate group had a risk reduction of 34 per cent, with a mortality of 25 per cent, compared with 34 per cent for those in the placebo group. Prazosin was no different from placebo. In about half the patients the aetiology of heart failure was CAD and in these the mortality on placebo was higher than the placebo group without coronary disease (see Figure 17.1). A benefit from hydralazine/nitrate therapy was still seen.

How can we interpret this study for clinical practice? The results give support to the concept that unloading (vasodilating) the heart is more rational than stimulating (inotropes) a myocardium that has already failed the body's intrinsic responses. However the study does not tell us how to do this other than by using the very high doses of isosorbide dinitrate combined with very high doses of hydralazine. Adverse effects were encountered frequently so that after six months, of those on placebo 84 per cent continued, on prazosin 75 per cent, and on hydralazine/isosorbide only 55 per cent were on full dosage. Interestingly 45 per cent of deaths were sudden. Does this mean that there may be, after all, a role for antiarrhythmics but only if combined with vasodilators? What happens beyond two years (though benefit was shown at three years the numbers were small)? Does this mean the end of the use of prazosin in heart failure or is its role to be in combination with nitrates? Careful scrutiny shows that the prazosin patients were significantly worse at entry—by keeping level with placebo did prazosin confer a benefit? Can this trial of moderate heart failure be extended to mild or severe heart failure? Can the results be extended to other vasodilators, eg, captopril?

Angiotensin-converting enzyme inhibitors (captopril, enalapril) are the subject of intensive study. There is no conclusive evidence on mortality in cases of mild to moderate heart failure but a pooling of trials points towards a reduction in mortality. The Consensus, a recent study of enalapril in severe heart failure (NYHA IV—breathless at rest) has shown that enalapril added to coventional therapy can reduce mortality and symptoms (The Consensus Trial Study Group, 'Effects of Enalapril on Mortality in Severe Congestive Heart Failure', *New Engl J Med* 1987, 316:1429–35). The improvement in mortality rate is due to a reduction in death from the progression of heart failure, sudden death not being influenced. The adverse effects caused by enalapril were hypotension, real insufficiency and potassium retention. In-patient monitoring and careful regular out-patient follow-up is therefore essential. The Consensus trial cannot directly be compared with the hydralazine/nitrate trial because the patients studied were completely different, but it does seem that at last heart failure patients have a real hope of a better quality of life for longer. The implication from both trials is that a combination of nitrate and angiotensin-converting enzyme inhibitors may extend the benefit, and trials are in progress. There should be no quarrel with the objective of improving the appalling prognosis and benefitting the quality of life. My interpretation is:

1   The vasodilator concept is the most promising.

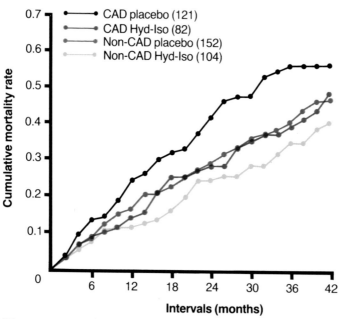

Figure 17.1 Cumulative mortality among patients with (n=203) and without (n=256) CAD treated with placebo or hydralazine plus isosorbide dinitrate (Hyd-Iso).[4]

2   Hydralazine and nitrates together are the only drugs currently known to improve prognosis in moderate heart failure.

3   Other drugs cannot be extrapolated; otherwise, prazosin would have been considered a reasonable alternative.

4   Prazosin may work in combination with nitrates and cannot be dismissed on the basis of this study.

5   Trials are needed with the other groups of drugs, and nitrates as monotherapy should be considered.

6   Where CAD is a cause of chronic heart failure, nitrates should be an early therapeutic option.

7   In severe heart failure enalapril or captopril should be initiated in hospital.

PATHOPHYSIOLOGY

Heart failure results in several compensatory mechanisms: the renin–angiotensin system is activated, the ventricle dilates and the sympathetic nervous system stimulates the heart and peripheral vessels. These mechanisms may be thought to be more appropriate as a response to loss of circulating blood volume and while helpful at first, they may actually increase myocardial workload at a time of myocardial failure. It is important therefore that before heart failure is treated the concepts and responses are understood, which means coming to terms with the terminology.

TERMINOLOGY AND REGULATION OF CARDIAC FAILURE

Cardiac output

This is the stroke volume (volume of blood ejected with each heart beat) multiplied by the heart rate:

$$CO = SV \times HR$$

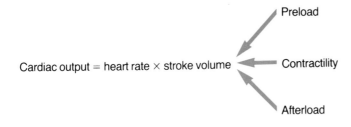

Preload

Contractility

Afterload

Cardiac output = heart rate × stroke volume

Figure 17.2   Three principal determinants of stroke volume.

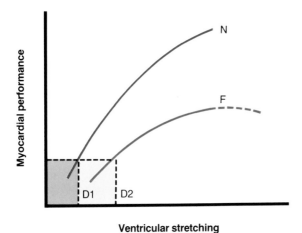

Myocardial performance

N

F

D1   D2

Ventricular stretching

Figure 17.3   Ventricular function curves. The normal heart (N) contrasts with the failing heart (F). (See text.)

As output falls the rate will rise usually due to responses from the sympathetic nervous system. However, three functions in addition to heart rate regulate the stroke volume and output—these being preload, afterload and contractility (see Figure 17.2).

Preload

Preload is the volume of blood present in the left ventricle at the end of diastole, ie, immediately before ejection. This could also be considered in terms of the degree of stretch experienced by the left ventricular muscle as a result of the volume of blood at the end of diastole. Starling[5] showed that the volume of ejected blood increases in response to myocardial stretching. This important compensatory mechanism helps to maintain cardiac output at or near normal levels even in quite advanced heart failure. In Figure 17.3, two ventricular curves are shown, one for a normal and one for a failing heart. Ventricular performance has been plotted against the volume of blood inside the ventricle at the end of diastole. Higher end-diastolic volumes result in greater stretching of the myocardium and a greater volume of blood is ejected. In heart failure the ventricular function curve is depressed because of a fall in contractility (change from N to F). Only in terminal heart failure is the curve of left ventricular function considered to be downsloping (the discontinued portion in line F).

For each unit increase in preload there should be a unit increase in output. This occurs to D1 in the normal heart but in the failing heart a greater increase in stretch results in a less significant increase in output (D2). Once a critical rise in stretch occurs the failing heart will be unable to respond and back pressure failure will occur.

While the horizontal axis relates to ventricular stretching, other terms may be used:

- LVEDP: left ventricular end-diastolic pressure (mmHg)
- LVFP: left ventricular filling pressure (mmHg)
- LVEDV: left ventricular end-diastolic volume (ml).

On the vertical axis, stroke work index (g.m/m^2) may replace myocardial performance.

Causes of increased preload

In heart failure preload is increased at rest which helps to maintain the resting cardiac output at normal or near normal levels. The mechanisms responsible for this are increased back pressure, increased venous tone, and salt and water retention (see Figure 17.4). Back pressure failure is one of the fundamental features of cardiac failure resulting in pulmonary oedema. Salt and water retention results from reduction in cardiac output influencing the renin production by the kidney (see Figure 17.5). Renin is increased secondary to diminished blood flow, and angiotensin is activated which increases aldosterone production. This promotes salt and water reabsorption by the kidney. Angiotensin II is a potent vasoconstrictor which increases peripheral resistance. This series of responses (retention of fluid and increasing resistance, ie, blood pressure) is more relevant to fluid loss rather than cardiac failure where it may add to the cardiac load, thereby being counterproductive.

The capacitance of the venous system is reduced in heart failure because of increased sympathetic tone. Eighty per cent of the blood volume may be in the venous capacitance vessels and sympathetic stimulation will cause venoconstriction, decreased pooling and increased venous return (preload). In addition sympathetic stimulation will also increase peripheral resistance (afterload).

Thus, while these responses increase myocardial stretching in attempting to maintain output, they also increase capillary pressure which is responsible for the congestion—

usually the most prominent feature of heart failure.

Afterload

Afterload is an expression of the force the heart muscle must generate to overcome the resistance to blood flow in the aorta and peripheral arteries. The resistance in the aorta is known as the *aortic impedance* and the resistance of the smaller vessels is known as the *peripheral resistance*. Afterload can therefore be seen as reflecting the sum of the two—the *total peripheral resistance* (TPR).

With increased venous return comes ventricular dilatation. This results in an increase in pressure which has to develop to eject a given volume of blood. This is the result of

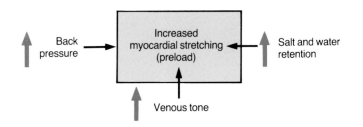

Figure 17.4 Factors affecting preload in heart failure.

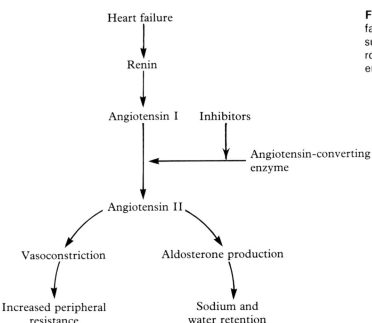

Figure 17.5 Effect of heart failure on renin release and the subsequent responses. The role of angiotensin-converting enzyme inhibitors is shown.

159

the Laplace principle which relates the tension in the myocardial fibre to the intracavity pressure and ventricular radius. Thus, afterload will be increased by increased preload and, of therapeutic importance, a reduction in preload will have secondary effects on reducing afterload. In Figure 17.6 the factors affecting afterload are summarized and Figure 17.7 relates afterload to the degree of failure.

Again it can be seen that the changes are designed more for hypovolaemia. Bloodflow is increased to the brain and coronary arteries at the expense of the splanchnic beds, peripheral muscles and kidneys. The patients may well have cold peripheries ('shut down') and be peripherally cyanosed.

Contractility

This refers to the force of ventricular contraction independent of loading, ie, it is intrinsic to the contractile proteins actin and myosin which are found in the thick and thin filaments of the myocardial sarcomere. An increase in sympathetic tone as well as increasing heart rate ($CO = SV \times HR$) also helps to maintain the contractile state of the failing heart, but at the expense of increased preload,

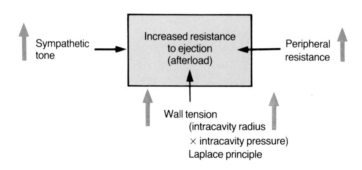

Figure 17.6 Factors affecting afterload in cardiac failure.

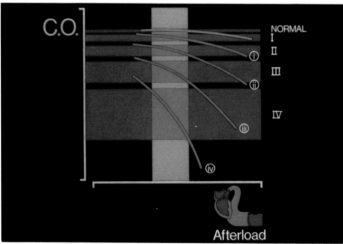

Figure 17.7 Effect of afterload. Decreased contractility or increased afterload result in depression of output and a move from the normal curve to the failure curves of the NHYA classification. C.O.=Cardiac output.

afterload and oxygen demand as a result of the increase in heart rate (remember also the coronary arteries fill in diastole).

Cardiac noradrenaline stores decrease with time in patients with heart failure[6] rendering them dependent on circulatory catecholamines. The higher the level the more severe the failure.[7] However, with prolonged stimulation may come a decrease in the numbers of active beta-adrenergic receptors ('down regulation') in the myocardium. This down regulation combined with decreased myocardial catecholamine content may lead to progressively reduced responsiveness to sympathetic stimulation.[8] Thus, longterm sympathetic responses may be as counterproductive as they are short-term.

SUMMARY

The primary determinants of cardiac function are:

- Preload
- Afterload
- Contractility
- Heart rate (and rhythm).

Cardiac status can be thought of as a chain with these four links; whichever is the weakest may lead to heart failure. In early failure when preload may be unchanged an increase in heart rate compensates and this may be an important early warning sign in a vulnerable patient. With *compensated* heart failure the preservation of output occurs as a result of the body's intrinsic abilities (increased sympathetic activity, ventricular dilatation and hypertrophy). *Decompensated* failure occurs when the prime mechanisms are inadequate.

When heart failure develops both preload and afterload will be increased. Increased preload helps to maintain cardiac output but is responsible for oedema (increased preload = back pressure failure = pulmonary congestion = dyspnoea). It also increases afterload by the Laplace effect. Increased afterload increases the work required to pump blood around the body and is liable to further reduce myocardial performance. Thus the pathophysiology of cardiac failure can be seen as a vicious circle where failure begets failure (see Figure 17.8). It is our purpose to break this circle.

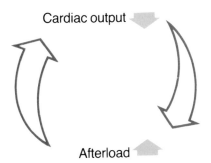

Cardiac output

Afterload

Figure 17.8 Vicious circle of heart failure.

SIGNS AND SYMPTOMS

The chapter on symptoms should be referred to (see page 29).

Breathlessness

This is the most common complaint usually reflecting a preload problem. It can vary from only minimal restriction to breathlessness at rest (see NYHA classification, page 41). Breathlessness when the patient is lying flat is known as orthopnoea, and paroxysmal nocturnal dyspnoea (PND) relates to gasping respiration, coughing and wheezing with occasionally frothy sputum, usually waking the patient. This reflects nocturnal absorption of fluid and increased preload at a time of decreased awareness, sleep. Patients should be asked how they sleep—do they use one, two or three pillows or do they sleep sitting in a chair for relief?

Fatigue and lethargy

These can be considered as afterload problems. Lack of cardiac output may interfere with cerebral flow (confusion, slowness, muddleheadedness) and skeletal perfusion (fatigue, heavy legs, 'everything an effort').

Oedema

Swollen ankles is the most frequent complaint, the problem being worse at the end of the day—'My shoes seem tight'. This follows a rise in right heart pressure which, if severe, can cause hepatic congestion and upper gastrointestinal engorgement. The patient may complain of right hypochondrial pain (tender swollen liver), anorexia, nausea or a bloated feeling. Older patients often do not complain until there is thigh and scrotal oedema with ascites.

EXAMINATION

In congestive cardiac failure the jugular venous pressure (JVP) may be raised (see Figure 17.9). This is best measured with the patient at 90 degrees, when the presence of any external or internal jugular venous filling above the sternal notch means raised pressure (using the external jugular vein is perfectly acceptable providing free fall occurs after finger pressure occlusion). The vein is best seen with a torch light at an angle to show it in relief. If the tricuspid valve is incompetent prominent CV waves will be seen and a pulsatile liver felt (remember it may be tender, too).

Along with a fall in output may come peripheral cyanosis, ankle oedema (see Figure 17.10), ascites (large abdomen, dull to percussion, usually tense), jaundice (hepatic congestion) and a wasted cachectic appearance. Invariably there is a sinus tachycardia with or without extrasystoles and in the more chronic cases atrial fibrillation is frequent. The blood pressure may be normal high or low depend-

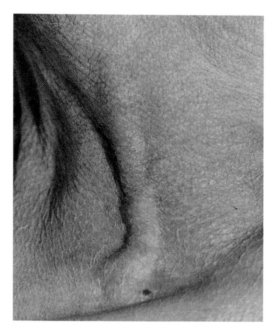

Figure 17.9   Rise of the JVP.

ing on the aetiology (eg, hypertension) and state of left ventricular function.

Cardiomegaly is frequent in chronic heart failure and III and/or IV sounds may be audible. Third sounds reflect a volume overloaded ventricle and IV sounds a pressure overloaded ventricle. Care must be taken to assess murmurs and judge their significance, eg, is the mitral incompetence the cause of the failure (when ischaemic it is usually loud, harsh, radiating to axilla and back with a thrill) or functional due to a dilated ring (soft, pansystolic, not usually radiating to the back)?

The lungs may be oedematous with basal crackles and bronchospasm and occasionally a pleural effusion will be present (no air entry, dull to percussion). This can be unilateral as well as bilateral.

Although this chapter is concerned with the treatment of the heart failure state because of muscle failure and CAD, it is important to consider other causes of heart failure and ask the following questions.

1 **Is there an underlying cardiac cause?**
    Look for evidence of valvar pathology, remembering that when cardiac output is low murmurs will be soft and should not be dismissed as 'functional' or 'insignificant' without objective assessment by chest x-ray examination and echocardiography.[9] Constrictive pericarditis still presents frequently enough after a liver biopsy to illustrate the need to be aware of other causes besides those that appear to be obvious.

2 **Is there a non-cardiac cause or iatrogenic origin?**
    Is there evidence of thyrotoxicosis, anaemia and severe infection (especially pneumonia in the elderly)? Has the patient been taking beta-blockers, cal-cium antagonists, non-steroidal anti-inflammatory agents or carbenoxalone?

3 **Is this really heart failure?**
    Many patients describe the tightness of angina as breathlessness. Is the patient anxious and hyperventilating?

INVESTIGATIONS

Chest x-ray examination

This should be routine and can be used to monitor therapy. If the transverse diameter of the heart is greater than 15.5 cm in the man and 14.5 cm in the woman there is cardiomegaly (see Figure 17.11). When the pulmonary venous pressure rises, first the upper zone veins become dilated—'upper zone blood vessel dilatation'. As the pulmonary pressure increases, usually above 20 mmHg, Kerley lines appear and finally at greater than 25 mmHg pulmonary oedema (see page 107).

The chest x-ray can also identify valvar calcification, suggest a left ventricular aneurysm (see page 110) or rarely pick up pericardial calcification (see Figure 17.12).

Electrocardiogram

While there are no specific ECG features of heart failure, the ECG is used to confirm the cardiac rhythm, assess the presence or absence of ventricular hypertrophy, and identify specific changes such as infarction or ischaemia.

Echocardiography

It is my routine policy to perform an echocardiogram on all patients undergoing therapy for chronic heart failure. While it may establish the diagnosis of a myopathic ventricle it also excludes significant suspected or unsuspected valvar pathology[9] which can be quantified with Doppler (see Figure 17.13). Echocardiography may identify a significant and operable left ventricular aneurysm as well as

163

intracavity thrombus. The presence of echocardiographic global left ventricular dysfunction will preclude the need for diagnostic angiography, and Doppler assessment of valvar incompetence will avoid unnecessary angiography to assess the functional significance of a murmur in the presence of severe left ventricular dysfunction.

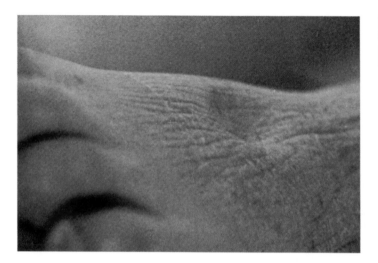

Figure 17.10 Ankle oedema. Often best judged by pressing above the ankle on the inside of the lower leg.

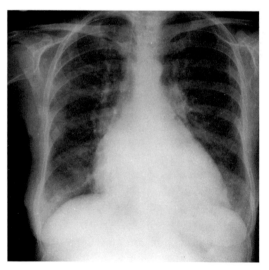

Figure 17.11 Cardiomegaly, upper zone blood diversion and Kerley lines.

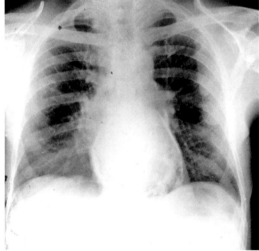

Figure 17.12 Pericardial calcification.

164

Angiography

This must be reserved for cases in which there is diagnostic doubt or uncertainty as to whether there is a mechanical problem that can be corrected. With the developments in echocardiography and colour flow Doppler (see Figure 17.14) angiography is likely to be necessary in only a small number of patients.[10]

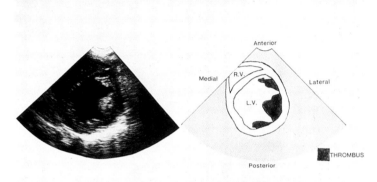

Figure 17.13
Echocardiogram showing global left ventricular dysfunction with thrombosis. RV=right ventricle; LV=left ventricle.

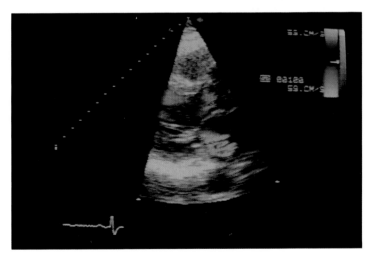

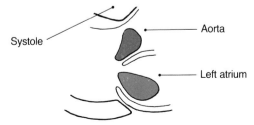

Figure 17.14 Colour flow Doppler evaluating mitral incompetence. Red coloured flow enters the aorta in systole with a blue coloured flow into the left atrium indicating mitral regurgitation.

165

MANAGEMENT

After removing any underlying cause (eg, aortic stenosis) and treating any precipitating factor (eg, arrhythmias) there remains the heart failure state, which is invariably due to left ventricular dysfunction. Treating the heart failure state will involve some or all of the following:

- Control of excessive preload
- Reduction of afterload
- Increased myocardial contractility.

	Sodium mg per 100g	Potassium mg per 100g
Bread		
Brown	550	210
White	540	100
Breakfast cereals		
Cornflakes	1160	99
Weetabix	360	420
Porridge	580	42
Drinks		
Coffee, instant	41	4000
Drinking chocolate	250	410
Leaf vegetables		
Spinach, boiled	120	490
Broccoli tops, boiled	6	220
Brussels sprouts, boiled	2	240
Cabbage (winter), boiled	4	160
Cauliflower, boiled	4	180
Celery, raw	140	280
Lettuce, raw	9	240
Root vegetables		
Carrots, boiled	50	87
Parsnips, boiled	4	290
Potatoes (new), boiled	41	330
Potatoes, chipped	12	1020
Peas (frozen), boiled	2	130
Peas (canned), garden	230	130
Beans (broad), boiled	20	230
Beans, baked and canned in tomato sauce	80	300
Beans, (runner), boiled	1	150
Fruit		
Blackberries	4	210
Raisins, dried	52	860
Bananas	1	350
Pears, fresh, eating	1	94
Strawberries	2	160
Plums, raw, eating	2	190
Apples	2	120
Oranges	3	200
Tomatoes, raw	3	290
Pineapple, fresh	2	250
canned	1	94
Grapefruit	1	230
Meat		
Roast chicken, meat only	81	310
Lamb chop, grilled, lean	72	320
Pork chop, grilled, lean	84	380
Rump steak, grilled, lean	55	380
Bacon, average lean rasher, grilled	2240	350
Pork sausage, grilled	1000	200
Fish		
Cod, fried in batter	100	370
Haddock, fried	180	350
Plaice, fried in crumbs	220	280
Scampi, fried	380	390

Table 17.1 Sodium and potassium content of everyday foods

166

General measures

To rest the heart we need to rest the individual. In severe heart failure bed rest is essential. However, some patients are more comfortable sitting in a chair by the bed and this is perfectly satisfactory. Passive or active leg exercises are recommended to prevent the development of deep venous thrombosis. With severe heart failure and gross peripheral oedema, however, early anticoagulation is recommended to prevent intraventricular clot as well as venous thrombosis. Patients should be allowed the use of the commode and when able should be allowed up to the toilet as this is less stressful physiologically and psychologically. A gentle laxative such as lactulose should be prescribed to avoid constipation (diuretics may dehydrate the bowels) and the adverse physiological effects of straining.

Smoking must be stopped or restricted to three cigarettes a day. At this point in severe heart failure the patient needs his maximum oxygen carrying capacity. Alcohol can be allowed in moderation but a high intake can depress contractility.[11]

Small meals are better tolerated and salt should be avoided in excess (2 g day or less). This means avoiding adding salt at the table and steering clear of sodium rich foods (Table 17.1). With the advent of powerful diuretics milder heart failure can usually be managed with a normal diet. Drugs with a high salt content (parenteral antibiotics, certain antacids) should be avoided, and those with the potential to retain salt and water (carbenoxolone and the non-steroidal anti-inflammatory agents) should either be avoided or used with caution. With stabilization of heart failure must come advice on weight and diet for longterm benefit in reducing cardiac work and oxygen demand.

Those living alone may need social support (home help, etc.) and should be allocated ground floor accommodation, not in a hilly environment. With the generally poor prognosis, attention to these details can have a major impact on the remaining quality of life.

DRUG THERAPY

Stimulation or unloading?

Stimulation (inotropy) is the policy of getting more out of the failing heart. Unloading (vasodilation) relies on manipulating the circulation to reduce the volume load on the heart and facilitate output. In patients where CAD is the cause of heart failure, attempts to make the heart work harder may have additional implications for the degree of ischaemia, making it worse by increasing oxygen demand at a time of decreased supply. Furthermore, improvement in exercise ability relates to improved (less) vasoconstriction which is a function of vasodilators rather than inotropes.[12] The failing heart, by virtue of the body's intrinsic responses, is functioning at near optimal power and further stimulation is akin to 'flogging a dead horse'.[13] While stimulating the failing heart with intravenous inotropes in severe heart failure may allow time to establish control with vasodilators (if the blood pressure will allow), it is usually only a temporary measure designed to buy time either to establish pharmaceutical control or to enable a heart transplant donor to be found. Improvement in exercise capacity without deleterious effects on the myocardium is the principal objective of therapy (it is too late for prevention) and this is the role of vasodilator therapy.[14]

Control of excessive preload

Increased preload with all its consequences is almost invariable in untreated heart failure. The aim of therapy is to reduce preload to levels which prevent tissue congestion or oedema. It must be remembered, however, that an excessive reduction in preload will cause the cardiac output to fall, and it is the presence of an increased preload which is necessary for vasodilators to work.[15] Look

167

now at Figure 17.15. As shown before (see Figure 17.3) patients with myocardial damage have a depressed left ventricular function curve. When the stroke volume falls (A–B) preload is increased because of fluid retention and venoconstriction (B–C). Increased levels of circulating catecholamines may increase contractility (C–F). Diuretics and venodilators reduce filling pressure (preload) without any significant effect on output (stroke volume). If the curve is flat, movement will be from C to D but too great a reduction will take the preload from D to E. At this point the curve is still rising, so drying out the patient too much will actually cause output to fall. Agents that reduce afterload or improve contractility result in movement from C to F, whereas adding preload reduction to afterload reduction obtains the best of both mechanisms; C to G (ie, less congestion, more output).

Successful management may become more difficult as heart failure worsens, with the problem of steering a course between hypovolaemia and a lower output on one hand and oedema on the other. Early use of vasodilators with periodic intravenous inotropic boosts may help here.

Diuretics

As excessive sodium and water retention are part of the compensatory response to cardiac failure so diuretics become a logical part of the management. In most instances they represent the mainstay of therapy. Care must be taken to tailor the diuretic dose to the individual patient's needs. Hospital admissions are too often caused by a carefully adjusted regime being suddenly altered, while in contrast many patients continue diuretics in too high a dosage, becoming dehydrated, dry-skinned and looking lethargic or 'washed out'.

When initiating therapy and adjusting

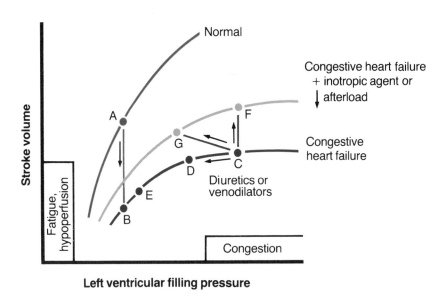

Figure 17.15 Effects of drug therapy on left ventricular performance in patients with congestive heart failure. (See text for discussion.)

diuretic dosage, frequent clinical assessment is required. Measurement of urea and electrolytes is particularly useful, with a rising urea pointing to over diuresis and a falling sodium to excessive fluid ingestion (waterlogged). It is also important to keep the potassium level above 3.5 mmol/l (3.5 mEq/l) particularly in patients taking digoxin. Longterm use of loop diuretics may lead to calcium and/or magnesium deficiency which should be monitored in patients on higher doses (over 160 mg frusemide daily).

Diuretics are principally preload reducers acting to reduce back pressure failure and relieve the symptom of dyspnoea. Their sites of action are shown in Figure 17.16.

THIAZIDES These act on the distal tubule of the kidney, interfering with sodium and water resorption. They are most effective in mild heart failure. Their action is gentler than the loop diuretics, beginning by 1 hour, peaking at 4 hours and being sustained over 10–12 hours. They are therefore less socially inconvenient and less likely to precipitate prostatic symptoms in the elderly man.

LOOP DIURETICS These are potent agents which when given intravenously are also powerful vasodilators.[16] They exert their main effects on the ascending limb of the loop of Henle with a weak effect on the convoluted tubule. They are rapid acting agents, effective intravenously in 5 minutes, orally in 1 hour, peaking within 2 hours, with a duration of action of 4–6 hours. Frusemide and bumetanide are the most widely used agents, being very effective either orally or intravenously. It is often forgotten that for patients who have never received diuretics 20 mg of frusemide is often enough, and that in patients with severe heart failure poor absorption necessitates the intravenous route. It should also be noted that thiazides and loop diuretics, by virtue of their different modes of action, can be used in combination for additive effects (eg, frusemide 80 mg plus bendrofluazide 5 mg daily). Occasionally when frusemide does not prove effective bumetamide will be and vice versa.

POTASSIUM SPARING AGENTS Spironolactone inhibits the effects of aldosterone in the distal tubule. It is especially useful when

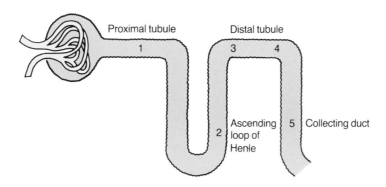

Figure 17.16 Sites of action of diuretics. Frusemide: 2, 1; bumetamide: 2,1; thiazides: 3; spironolactone, triamterene and amiloride: 4, 5.

hepatic congestion leads to secondary hyper-aldosteronism. It antagonizes potassium excretion and therefore represents a useful combination with loop or thiazide diuretics. The onset of action, however, is 48–72 hours so it is not an immediate remedy for hypokalaemia. In patients with reduced renal function the possibility of hyperkalaemia should be remembered. The major limitation to therapy in men is gynaecomastia, which may be painful.

Amiloride and triamterene exert potassium sparing effects independent of aldosterone and they do not lead to gynaecomastia. I use spironolactone 50 mg/40 mg of frusemide with a usual maximum of 100 mg daily and amiloride 5 mg/40 mg of frusemide with a maximum of 10 mg daily. Further doses of frusemide can be used and only rarely is more potassium sparing agent needed.

Choice of diuretic

As in mild heart failure thiazides often suffice, it is here where they form primary therapy. For patients with an adequate diet 5 mg of bendrofluazide together with advice on potassium-containing foods may be all that is needed (see Table 17.1). When digoxin is coprescribed or the diet is variable (eg, with the elderly or unemployed) a potassium sparing combination is preferred. I use hydrochlorothiazide 25 mg plus triamterene 50 mg once or twice daily, or spironolactone 50 mg plus hydroflumethiazide 50 mg once, twice or half strength daily. I rarely use amiloride hydrochloride 5 mg, hydrochorothiazide 50 mg because of an unpredictable tendency to hyponatraemia, particularly in the elderly.

I only use potassium supplements for the immediate treatment of hypokalaemia and not as longterm agents, and prefer effervescent potassium to slow release agents. Avoid large tablets which can stick in the elderly's oesophagus because of poor motility or lodge where an enlarged left atrium presses back onto the oesophagus.

170

For more severe heart failure use loop diuretics again with potassium sparing agents. Severe cases (oedema to the knees, raised JVP, big liver) may have bowel oedema and poor oral absorption so a short course of intravenous frusemide is indicated. When the failure is controlled dosage can often be decreased. It is difficult to be precise about dosage because of the individual needs of the patient. In general practice, if breathlessness continues in spite of thiazides (eg, triamterine 50 mg, hydrochlorothiazide twice daily), I would change to frusemide 40 mg plus amiloride 5 mg or frusemide 40 mg plus triamterene 50 mg once or twice daily, but any higher dose needs hospital assessment.

Loop diuretics should not be used with cephalosporins because of nephrotoxicity, and in the mentally ill lithium levels may be increased. It should also be remembered that in very high doses ototoxicity occurs (ask the patient about tinnitus and deafness).

Adverse effects

Inappropriate usage remains the greatest cause of drug-induced side-effects and for many patients diuretics are pushed too hard when alternatives should be added (see Figure 17.15).

HYPOKALAEMIA This can be prevented by dietary advice and, if needed, by using potassium sparing agents. It is important to remember the risks of hyperkalaemia when renal function is reduced and with the wider use of angiotensin-converting enzyme inhibitors, hyperkalaemia may rapidly result if potassium sparing agents are coprescribed.

HYPONATRAEMIA This is often the problem in the grossly oedematous patient who appears refractory to diuretic therapy. Admission to hospital is essential and management surrounds fluid restriction (1000–1500 cc/day or less), diuretic reduction and the use of vasodilators and inotropes.

In the elderly in particular, especially when amiloride is involved, diuretic-induced hyponatraemia may occur and present as weakness, nausea and confusion. It may be necessary to provide added sodium but in the presence of severe heart failure this will be a difficult and dangerous option to be pursued only as a last resort.[17] When corrected, a change in diuretic is essential with a move away from the distally acting agents (amiloride, triamterene).

HYPERURICAEMIA Diuretics decrease the renal clearance of uric acid, raise urate levels and may therefore either exacerbate or precipitate gout. Acute attacks require treatment with specific anti-inflammatory agents such as indomethacin. This may promote sodium and water retention, however, rendering the diuretic less effective. Colchicine is an alternative. In the longterm those vulnerable should receive allopurinol.

GLUCOSE INTOLERANCE This needs to be remembered in older patients and diabetics whose control may be lost. Dietary and drug therapy will be needed when glucose intolerance persists as a result of anti-failure therapy because in most patients the anti-failure therapy will be life-long. Sometimes hyperglycaemia resolves when associated hypokalaemia is corrected.

Diuretic resistance

The need for the intravenous route when heart failure is severe has already been discussed. Metolazone is dramatically effective in some resistant patients. I use 5–10 mg daily and because of the scale of the effect (one of my patients lost 12 kg (26 lb) in 12 hours) fluid monitoring must be carefully done in case of too rapid an action.[18] The onset of action is 1 hour with peak effect at 4 hours and duration of action up to 48 hours. When oral frusemide is not totally effective alone, say at 80 mg twice daily, rather than increasing the dose, adding in bendrofluazide 5 or 10 mg may be nearly as effective as metolazone but less dramatic.

Monitoring effect

Daily weights are the most reliable, with 1 kg (2.20 lb) equivalent to 1 litre. A weight change each day of greater than 0.5 kg (1.10 lb) is the objective of diuretic therapy. Excessive weight loss points to over diuresis and weight gain to ineffective therapy.

Vasodilators

Vasodilators can be used to reduce preload by dilating venous capacitance vessels or afterload by dilating aterioles.[19] Patients whose symptoms reflect increased preload (venous congestion) should respond better to a venodilator, while patients with depressed left ventricular function and symptoms of low output should respond better to an arteriolar dilator. However, as the two conditions must often go together a drug with both properties—a balanced vasodilator, or a mixture of venous and arterial dilators—should be the most effective. Table 17.2 lists the important oral and intravenous vasodilators.

In the past vasodilators tended to be reserved for the more severe cases of heart failure but their earlier use is likely to lead to lower diuretic dosage and an improved quality of life. In this way it may be possible to switch from loop to thiazide diuretics.[20]

Nitrates

These are the main preload reducers.[21] They are especially useful in ischaemic heart failure when pain may coexist. They may be given orally, topically, intravenously and via the mucous membranes. Most studies have been with isosorbide dinitrate[22] but this is subject to first pass metabolism in the liver, leading to variable blood levels of the active metabolite isosorbide 5 mononitrate (see page 59). Isosorbide 5 mononitrate (ISMN) is therefore to be preferred. Topical nitrates may be useful

171

for nocturnal breathlessness,[23] leading to a regime of ISMN 20 or 40 mg twice daily with a fresh patch at night. Nitrates are most effective in patients with pulmonary congestion and a normal or slightly reduced cardiac output. They can be used in combination with other vasodilators and intravenously in the acute setting when mitral regurgitation can also be reduced.

Side-effects include headaches, flushing, and occasionally tachycardia. Occasionally hypotension occurs and very rarely methaemaglobinaemia. Tolerance may be a problem but the recent mortality trial suggests otherwise.[4] It is always difficult to distinguish tolerance (decreased effect with time) from disease progression.[22]

In the ischaemic patient with heart failure, nitrates can be introduced after thiazide diuretics. It must be remembered that all vasodilators need raised preload to be effective, so the patient must not be overdiurised before he is started.

Afterload reduction
Drugs that reduce afterload will increase cardiac output (see Figure 17.7). The major limitation to their use is hypotension and they are not recommended if the systolic blood pressure is below 90 mmHg. I prefer a systolic pressure of 100 mmHg or greater but in severe failure I sometimes have little room to manoeuvre and very cautiously attempt therapy below 100 mmHg but above 90 mmHg. Afterload reducers are most effective when the output is decreased and the preload normal or raised. In the latter case combination with nitrates may give an additive effect.[24]

Most patients prescribed vasodilator drugs gain considerable symptomatic relief, although controversy remains as to whether the beneficial effects persist with time.[25] There is some doubt about whether a sustained increase in exercise tolerance takes place, but again it is difficult to distinguish drug effects from failures because of natural disease progression.

Prazosin
Prazosin is a balanced vasodilator which reduces both preload and afterload. It acts by blocking postsynaptic alpha receptors. Postural hypotension occurs but is unlikely when therapy starts with a low dose of 0.5 mg tds.

Table 17.2 Vasodilators used in the treatment of heart failure

Agent	Site of action Arterial	Venous	Mode of administration	Duration of action
Nitroglycerin	+	+ +	Sublingual, intravenous, topical	Minutes to hours
Isosorbide dinitrate	+	+ +	Sublingual, oral, intravenous	Minutes to hours
Isosorbide mononitrate	+	+ +	Oral	Hours
Nitroprusside	+ +	+ +	Intravenous	Minutes
Prazosin	+ +	+ +	Oral	Hours
Hydralazine	+ +	+	Oral	Hours
Captopril	+ +	+	Oral	Hours
Enalapril	+ +	+	Oral	Hours

The dose should be titrated at weekly intervals until optimum dose is achieved. The average dose is 2 mg tds but 5 mg or 10 mg bid may be needed. Prazosin has been found to be effective, particularly in combination with a regime including spironolactone.[20] Others, however, have shown tachyphylaxis despite an initially favourable response.[24,26] Tolerance can be circumvented by dosage manipulation, a temporary increase in diuretics or bed rest, but clinical and haemodynamic benefit persists in only 30 to 40 per cent of patients. It must be said that at present the place of prazosin in heart failure is unclear; its use is decreasing and with the disappointing lack of effect on mortality this is unlikely to be reversed. Concern remains that its role is not fully defined and before it is abandoned further assessments are needed, particularly of its use in combination with nitrates.

Hydralazine

Hydralazine is a direct smooth muscle relaxant which results in a potent arterial dilator action. Renal and limb blood flow increase and a sustained action on cardiac output has been demonstrated. Its use as a single agent and in combination with nitrates is well documented.[27,28] While tolerance has been recorded this may be less likely when combined with nitrates.[29]

Oral hydralazine in heart failure does not usually lead to a significant reflex tachycardia, probably because the sympathetic nervous system is fully active or exhausted. The drug is vulnerable to hepatic metabolism with a bioavailability of 25–55 per cent. Dosage needed for effect is usually 200 mg daily or greater. It is especially useful in reducing the regurgitant fraction of mitral or aortic incompetence. With higher doses comes the risk of the lupus syndrome. If high doses are being used (> 200 mg daily) the acetylator status should be recorded and, if slow, dosages reduced. Regular monitoring of antinuclear antibodies (three monthly) is recommended

with high dosage. Other adverse effects include precipitation of angina in those with severe coronary disease (less likely when combined with a nitrate), a severe headache and postural hypotension.

I mainly use this drug with a nitrate, beginning at 25 mg tds and increasing to 50 mg tds or, rarely, 100 mg tds. Its principal benefit is exerted when cardiac output is decreased.

Angiotensin-converting enzyme inhibitors

Angiotensin-converting enzyme inhibition is an area of intensive activity. These drugs have many desirable properties for the management of heart failure. They act by interfering with the renin–angiotensin system (see Figure 17.5). They reduce aldosterone production (a diuretic effect) and act as vasodilators, principally arteriolar. Two agents are available: captopril and enalapril. Trials of both have shown benefit in longterm treatment with improved symptoms, exercise duration and haemodynamics.[30,31] Mortality has been reduced by enalapril in severe heart failure (p 156), and captopril.[32]

These drugs are effective in severe and moderate heart failure and may work when other agents fail. The most frequent side-effect is hypotension and the drug must not be introduced in the presence of over diuresis. The differences between the drugs surround dosage, with captopril being a twice or thrice daily drug and enalapril a once daily agent. With captopril, occasional severe hypotension has been recorded after the first dose,[33] which has led to the sensible recommendation that this should be 6.25 mg, given with the patient supine and preferably in hospital. This hypotensive syncope coincides with a rapid fall in angiotensin II levels 30–45 minutes after dosage.[33] Enalapril exerts similar effects but 2–4 hours after dosage because of the delay in its conversion to the active metabolite enalaprilat.[34] It is clear that patients receiving these drugs should be under hospital supervision when the initial *low* dose is given. The Committee on Safety of Medicine in May 1986 recommended enalapril be always initiated in hospital at 2.5 mg. Cessation of diuretics beforehand is recommended but this does not always prevent syncope.[33] In some cases severe or prolonged hypotension has led to neurological deficit and renal failure. In others renal failure may be related to lowered filtration pressure and seems more common with enalapril. Other adverse effects include rashes, taste disturbances and haematological changes but these tend to be over-emphasized and perhaps reflect the initial use of too high a dosage in the early development of the drugs.[35]

Clinical use

Captopril has the safer profile in heart failure. The more prolonged action of enalapril may lead to a more prolonged hypotensive effect leading to a great chance of renal insufficiency.[36] Captopril should be reserved for hospital use, begun only in patients with adequate preload, commenced at 6.25 mg in the evening followed by 6.25 mg bid or tds for 24 hours. It can then be titrated to 12.5 mg bid or tds and to 25 mg bid or tds at 48 hour intervals, carefully monitoring blood pressure response. Always remember that potent diuretics combined with angiotensin-converting enzyme inhibitors can impair renal function and appropriate serial electrolyte checks must be taken. Captopril can be combined with nitrates.

Nifedipine

Calcium is fundamental to cardiac contraction. The argument for using nifedipine is that the afterload reducing effects will offset the potential for cardiac depression as a result of antagonizing calcium channels in the myocardium.[37] Effects are bound to be unpredictable, depending on the contractile state. It is fraught with avoidable risks not present with

174

other agents and it is bewildering that it is used at all in heart failure.

INOTROPIC AGENTS

In the management of chronic heart failure the only oral agent we currently have for longterm use is digoxin.

Cardiac glycosides

ATRIAL FIBRILLATION Digitalis is effective when heart failure is associated with atrial fibrillation. It stimulates the myocardium while depressing sinus rate and atrioventricular nodal function. The principal mechanisms of action are inhibition of sodium–potassium–adenosine–triphosphatase[38] and increased vagal activity.[39] Thus it slows the ventricular response in supraventricular tachyarrhythmias, prolongs diastole and improves output. Withering[40] noted a diuretic effect which is thought to represent a direct action on the renal tubules rather than a secondary response to increased output. When the ventricular response is greater than 100 beats/minute (measured at the apex or by ECG) digoxin should be started to try to get the rate below 100. Routine oral digitalization (day one 0.5 mg tds, day two 0.25 mg bid, day three and subsequently 0.25 mg om) is all that is usually necessary. If the blood urea is greater than 8 mmol/l (48 mg/100 ml) or the age over seventy all doses are halved after the first day loading dose.

If the ventricular rate is not controlled and signs of digoxin toxicity become evident then, in the setting of heart failure, amiodarone is the only agent which does not have a significant negative inotropic action. It does, however, increase plasma digoxin concentrations.[41] The recommendation is to withhold digoxin for 48 hours and then reintroduce at half dose combined with amiodarone 200 mg daily. Persistently rapid ventricular responses with no continuing failure should raise the suspicion of hyperthyroidism.

SINUS RHYTHM The role of digitalis in heart failure and sinus rhythm is controversial. There is a positive inotropic action acutely but over two to three months the effectiveness is disputed.[42,43] Reviewing the literature[43-45] some authors have concluded that it is not known whether cardiac glycosides exert a sustained and useful effect in chronic heart failure with sinus rhythm.[44,45] Furthermore, most patients in sinus rhythm with heart failure can have their maintenance therapy with digoxin discontinued without deterioration.[46] However, in one study fourteen of twenty-five patients deteriorated when placebo replaced digoxin but those who responded to digoxin had more severe failure and a III heart sound.[47] Diuretic dose was low in this study, so perhaps just increasing frusemide would have been as effective.

In clinical practice it can be said that, in acute heart failure, the first approach is diuretics and vasodilators. Digoxin may be successful as a third option if response is incomplete. If control is established it should be maintained for two to three months. If other agents are used optimally digoxin can be carefully withdrawn, and most patients will not deteriorate. A few, perhaps the more severe, may, when it should be reintroduced.

Glycosides available

DIGOXIN This is the agent of choice with the shortest half-life rendering management of toxicity easier. It is excreted by the kidneys with a half-life of 36 hours. Clearance is linearly related to creatinine clearance and the half-life can extend to four days with renal impairment. The elderly are prone to toxicity because of the age-related fall-off in renal function.[48] Hyperthyroidism increases clearance; hypothyroidism decreases it.[49]

After digitalization maintenance is usually 0.25 mg daily below sixty-five to seventy years and 0.0625–0.125 mg daily above.

MEDIGOXIN This is beta-methyl digoxin which is absorbed more readily from the gut than digoxin. The half-life is 60 hours so the toxic effects may be prolonged.

DIGITOXIN This is fully absorbed after oral administration. It is metabolized by the liver and excreted in the bile. With 90 per cent protein binding, the half-life is extended to five days with normal hepatic function. Although some prefer to use it in renal failure, the half-life renders toxicity management difficult.[50]

Toxicity One of the main reasons for re-evaluating the role of digoxin in heart failure is the narrow line between benefit and toxicity. Intoxication may occur when excretion is compromised or when excess is administered by prescription or overdose (suicide).

Toxicity of digoxin may occur with age, renal failure, hypokalaemia, anoxia, hypercalcaemia, hypomagnesaemia and hypothyroidism. Drug interactions likely to raise digoxin concentrations include spironolactone, triamterene, quinidine, verapamil, amiodarone and nifedipine.[43,51]

The signs and symptoms of toxicity are well known with anorexia, nausea and vomiting the most frequent.[52,53] Brady and tachyarrhythmias are more frequent with associated hypokalaemia but yellow vision is rare (teichopsia).

Digoxin toxicity may occur with raised serum concentrations but when the potassium is low the toxic levels may be in the so-called therapeutic range.[54] Cardiac manifestations of toxicity include ventricular bigeminy ('coupling') (see Figure 17.17), atrial tachycardia, heart block and ventricular tachycardia or fibrillation. Virtually any arrhythmia can be allocated to digoxin toxicity.

In most cases the patient complains of a loss of appetite, nausea or vomiting. Less frequently adverse effects of fatigue, headache, facial pain, and gynaecomastia occur. Measuring serum digoxin levels should occur with a simultaneous potassium level. If the potassium is normal, toxicity is unlikely with plasma digoxin below 2.5 nmol/l (2 ng/ml), whereas toxicity is almost certain above 5 nmol/l (4 ng/ml). When the potassium is below 3.5 mmol/l, toxicity may occur in the normal range of 1.3–2.5 nmol/l. Blood should be assayed 6–8 hours after the last oral dose.

In the clinical setting it is best to stop therapy if nausea develops. If the symptoms resolve, digoxin is reintroduced at half dosage after first establishing if it is really necessary and excluding any precipitating causes. With more complex manifestations of toxicity serum estimations are recommended.

Treatment of toxicity means stopping digoxin and, where applicable, correcting a low potassium level orally if mild, or intravenously if severe. (Do not forget to check magnesium also.) Arrhythmias should be managed with appropriate agents (eg, lignocaine or procainamide for ventricular problems, pacing for heart block or overdrive for resistant ventricular tachycardia, beta-blockers for supraventricular problems). If dc shocks are necessary, low energy should be used initially (25–50 joules).[55]

Digoxin-specific antibodies have been used in life-threatening cases with twenty-one of twenty-six patients surviving.[56] These are now available (Digibind–digoxin-specific antibody fragments) and should be thought of in severe cases (consult the Poisons Information Service).

Digoxin levels on maintenance therapy need not be measured routinely but can be of use when therapeutic responses are not as predicted, and when a multitude of complaints renders it impossible to assess the clinical implications of nausea or vomiting.

Other inotropic agents

These are mainly available intravenously. Dopamine or dobutamine can be used occasionally in severe chronic heart failure, in bursts for 24 hours to allow time to gain or regain control with diuretics and vasodilators.[57]

Dopamine and dobutamine have positive inotropic actions, with dopamine in low dosage (<5 µg/kg per minute) increasing renal sodium excretion.[58] Both are sympathomimetic amines and may accelerate the heart, increasing oxygen demand which could be

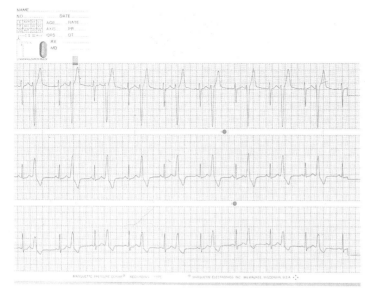

Figure 17.17 Ventricular bigeminy of digoxin toxicity.

disadvantageous in the presence of CAD. They are also potentially arrhythmogenic. Use of these agents is outlined in the section on acute heart failure (see page 108). Dopamine up to 5 µg/kg per minute can be used to avoid stimulation of peripheral alpha receptors which will lead to vasoconstriction and increased afterload and this can be combined with dobutamine titrated to effect (range 2.5–40 µg/kg per minute).

Oral agents exist which stimulate beta adrenoceptors. However, longterm administration will be expected to result in diminishing effects because of down regulation of the beta receptors[58] and of course this aspect of therapy is not physiologically sound on the background of the pathophysiology of heart failure. There is no evidence of longterm benefit from prenalterol, pirbuterol, or salbutamol.[42,59]

Non-cardiac glycoside, non-catecholamine inotropic agents being evaluated are amrinone and milrinone. They are vasodilators as well as inotropes. Oral amrinone has a high incidence of adverse effects and investigation has halted. Milrinone has fewer side-effects but the initial improvements have not been translated into longterm benefit and survival remains very poor.[60] In a comprehensive review of inotropes,[60] vasodilators are considered a more appropriate step than new inotropes in the context of continuing heart failure despite dietary therapy, digitalis and diuretics.

Beta-blockade

Several studies exist evaluating beta-blockade in heart failure. Results are conflicting and have been reviewed.[61] At present studies are small and there is a need for a large randomized trial with clear, well defined entry criteria and dosage. There does appear to be a group who would benefit, but trying to characterize this group is difficult. The theoretical benefit is derived from increased energy supply, improved diastolic relaxation, inhibition of sympathetically mediated vasoconstriction

and necrosis and 'up regulation' of the beta receptors. The potential for disaster is, however, obvious.[62] Beta-blockade must therefore currently only be used in a strictly controlled hospital environment in patients stabilized on vasodilators and diuretics.

Xamoterol

This cardioselective beta-partial agonist may be of value. When sympathetic tone is high the drug is a beta antagonist and when low (at rest or on mild exercise) a beta agonist. Its potential use for heart failure associated with angina is considerable if the idea translates into clinical benefit.[63] It may have the potential to 'up-regulate' beta receptors without too great a haemodynamic risk. Early results look promising and its potential in combination with vasodilators is considerable.

OTHER FORMS OF TREATMENT

Ultrafiltration and haemofiltration

These are complex expensive procedures to be considered only when a surgical option is possible for refractory heart failure, ie, they may buy time for transplantation or allow sufficient restoration of haemodynamic status to facilitate cardiac surgery.[64]

Surgery

Coronary artery bypass surgery may be of benefit when ischaemia leads to heart failure but ventricular function remains preserved when the condition is stabilized.[65] It will be of benefit when mechanical lesions are present and residual left ventricular function is adequate. In chronic heart failure because of myocardial loss, no benefit is recorded for surgery when the symptom limitation is failure.

Transplantation

Cardiac transplantation is the last option for a small number of patients. Immunosuppres-

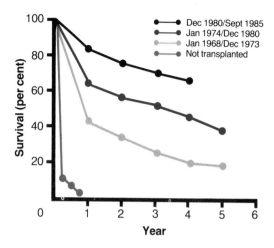

Legend:
- Dec 1980/Sept 1985
- Jan 1974/Dec 1980
- Jan 1968/Dec 1973
- Not transplanted

Figure 17.18 Survival with and without heart transplantation.

sive therapy remains imperfect and accelerated atheroma in the coronary arteries of the donor heart a major problem. The latest figures (see Figure 17.18) show a one-year survival of 85 per cent but the late five-year survival appears to be 66 per cent, with significant atherosclerois occurring in 40 per cent (see Figure 17.19) irrespective of whether or not the transplant was for coronary disease.[66]

Transplantation can be considered a reasonable option for patients who are less than fifty-five years of age, who have strong psychological[67] and social backgrounds and who understand that it may need repeating on several occasions. It is for most an expensive palliative but hard to deny to the young disabled heart failure patient who may be restored to a normal active (though perhaps temporary) life. While awaiting transplantation, mechanical assistance can preserve life until a donor is found.

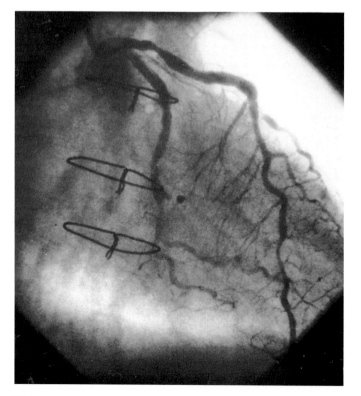

Figure 17.19 Advanced atheroma in a transplanted heart two years after insertion.

178

- Chronic heart failure implies that all correctable causes have been removed.

- Echocardiography is important in establishing that no occult surgical lesions exist and that muscle failure is the primary problem.

- Mild failure usually responds to diuretics and diet. Nitrates may be added before high doses of diuretics are used.

- Moderate failure requires loop diuretics, and vasodilators should be added above frusemide 40 mg.

- All vasodilators need preload and therefore the patient must not be over diuresed before treatment starts.

- Diuretics must be monitored with urea, and electrolytes and potassium sparing agents are preferable.

- If the output is adequate nitrates alone may help but if the output is reduced, afterload-reducing agents are needed (eg, hydralazine, captopril).

- Afterload reduction should begin in hospital.

- Captopril should be used without potassium sparing diuretics at first.

- Digoxin is essential with atrial fibrillation. Control may be helped with amiodarone.

- Digoxin in sinus rhythm is recommended when diuretics and vasodilators are not totally effective. After two to three months of stabilization it can cautiously be withdrawn.

- In severe heart failure anticoagulation may prevent embolization and venous thrombosis.

- No oral inotropic agents other than digoxin are available but periodic intravenous bursts of dopamine or dobutamine may reverse a desperate situation.

- Cardiac transplantation is an option for those under fifty-five years of age. Artificial assist devices can be used until a donor is found.

- Hydralazine and isosorbide dinitrate or angiotensin-converting enzyme inhibitors when added to digoxin and diuretics provide the only regimes known to reduce mortality.

18
Chest pain with normal coronary arteries

BACKGROUND

By definition this is a problem occurring after angiography. The patient has been investigated for chest pain believed to be of cardiac origin but atheroma has not been shown in the coronary tree. The incidence of the problem varies from 10–30 per cent[1,2] and must depend to some extent on whether noninvasive screening has been used to select those who do not need invasive procedures. Noninvasive screening in an atypical and typical chest pain population may still point to ischaemia, however, and abnormal thallium scans and changes in myocardial lactate metabolism on atrial pacing still occur in the presence of normal coronary arteriograms[3,4] (see Figure 18.1).

The prognosis is favourable with subsequent myocardial infarction and mortality not being increased above that in the population at large when measured ten years after angiography.[5] Unfortunately while the prognosis for survival is favourable, between 20 and 80 per cent of patients continue to complain of chest pain and suffer considerable functional disability after arteriography.[6–8] Repeated hospitalization or attendances for chest pain and continued cardiac medication, with between 30 and 50 per cent unable to work, identifies the major social and economic consequences.[9,10] With this somewhat awkward group to manage, the question remains what to do next, if anything.

AETIOLOGY

Coronary artery spasm (see page 77), cardio-myopathy,[11] small vessel disease[12] and defects of oxyhaemoglobin dissociation[13] have been suggested but only spasm is proven.[14] It is also well known that typical and atypical chest pains can occur in the presence of hypertension with normal coronary arteries and when mitral valve prolapse is present.[15]

There is no doubt, however, that the principal differential diagnosis rests between musculoskeletal pain, oesophageal pain,[16] hyperventilation syndrome and psychiatric morbidity.[17]

Oesophageal pain

The prevalence of oesophageal disease in patients with normal coronary arteries is reported to be between 17 and 100 per cent.[18] Although convinced of the cardiac diagnosis beforehand, retaking the history would appear to be the first sensible move. Oesophageal pain is typically brought on by stooping, may occur after eating or be associated with reflux. It is frequently worse when the patient is lying down and relieved by sitting up or standing. Although some authors propose vigorous testing to exclude oesophageal symptoms[19] others point out that abnormalities of the oesophagus can occur in the presence of coronary artery disease (CAD) and are not necessarily related to chest pain.[20,21]

Oesophageal pain may be secondary to simple reflux oesophagitis, spasm, or rarer motility disorders. A barium meal will demonstrate motility, spasm, and reflux, and endoscopy identify inflammation or ulcers. Acid perfusion can precipitate pain but should be done with a simultaneous ECG because of linked pain[21] and the known adverse effects on effort angina.[22] Oesophageal manometry is not widely available nor does it appear to clarify the diagnosis.[19-21]

From a practical point of view it seems reasonable to investigate the oesophagus in patients whose pain is brought on by stooping and eating, who experience reflux and get

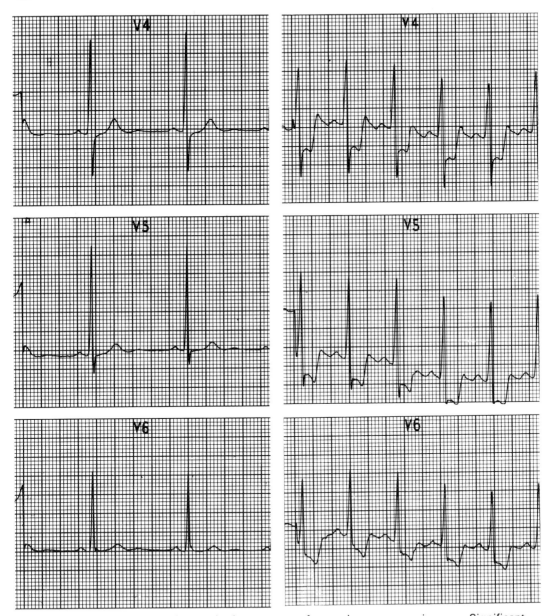

Figure 18.1 Abnormal exercise ECG in the presence of normal coronary angiograms. Significant ST depression (right) is shown compared with the resting trace (left). The patient had the angiogram repeated three times because of disbelief. He is alive, well and symptom-free twelve years later.

relief by standing, and taking antacids. A barium meal may establish the diagnosis and if any doubt remains an acid perfusion test can be done. Treatment can then be instituted (diet, antacids, antispasm agents) to relieve symptoms. There is not sufficient evidence available to justify extensive oesophageal function studies in those who have no symptoms to suggest a gastrointestinal problem.

Musculoskeletal pain

This is discussed in the chapter on symptoms. Here it is mentioned in the context of going back to the patient to retake the history. Can the pain be reproduced by pressure? Can the patient point to it? Is it positional? Is the tightness worse on deep breathing (pectoral spasm to stop movement caused by joint or root pain)? Can the patient walk around with it? Is it continuous? There is no shame in getting it wrong and needing an angiogram to identify musculoskeletal pain—as long as we are honest enough to go back and help the patient with the cause of the symptoms (eg, analgesia, physiotherapy).

Hyperventilation and psychiatric morbidity

In our department a prospective study using standardized measures of psychiatric and social morbidity was carried out, and a high rate of neurotic symptoms was found in patients without significant CAD. In particular, there was a relationship between symptoms of anxiety and panic, respiratory complaints and low levels of end-tidal pCO_2.[17] Half of the patients had phobic complaints and 11 per cent satisfied the criteria for agorophobia.[23] A prospective study confirmed the association between psychosocial morbidity and continued complaints of chest pain (40 per cent at one year).[8] More detailed laboratory investigations have confirmed our clinical impression that hyperventilation is an important pathophysiological mechanism responsible for the diverse symptomatology in a

182

subgroup of patients,[24] and it may even induce coronary artery spasm and myocardial damage.[25]

Making the diagnosis of hyperventilation relies on the history (atypical dyspnoea, air hunger, phobic symptoms, sighing, gasping, nocturnal breathlessness). Look at the patient—he may sigh, the upper thorax move excessively or he may pant obviously and frequently. The patient may have a sinus tachycardia, sweat easily, exhibit wheezing and chest wall tenderness. Hyperventilating patients are not usually able to hold their breath for 30 seconds. A forced hyperventilation test can be done at the bedside (see Table 18.1). A more invasive approach is to measure arterial or end-tidal pCO_2, which is abnormal below 30 mmHg and after forced hyperventilation should be back to normal in 3 minutes.

Management begins with explanation and reassurance. Drugs should be stopped and a normal lifestyle encouraged. Rebreathing from a paper bag should be taught. For many this is not enough and exercises are needed to educate the patients away from thoracic and towards diaphragmatic breathing at eight to twelve breaths per minute. Physiotherapists provide this service in outpatients and the patients practice 30 minutes each day. Inpatient therapy is recommended for the severe cases. Cardioselective beta-blockade can be used to reduce sympathetically mediated symptoms of palpitations, trembling and sweating and surprisingly high doses are frequently needed, eg, atenolol 100 or 200 mg a day (one patient needed 300 mg bid) and metoprolol 50–200 mg bid. Major psychiatric symptoms need referral to a specialist.

MANAGEMENT STRATEGY

The majority of patients with angina and normal coronary arteries have psychological factors to explain their symptoms rather than cardiac disease. I have changed my approach substantially from invasive[3,11] to noninva-

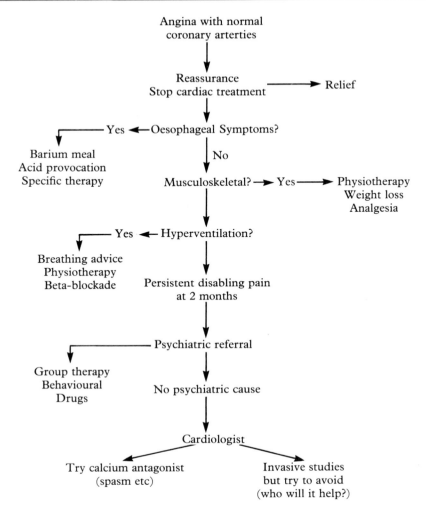

Figure 18.2 Management strategy for angina with normal coronary arteries.

sive.[8,17] I began several projects[8,17] because of the problem of telling an individual person he was normal and yet advising more invasive cardiac tests. Others still believe an investigative approach is justified to document coronary artery spasm and decrements in coronary reserve.[26] But as these form a relatively minor part of the problem it seems a rather invasive and expensive way of chasing scientific ideals.

A cardiac invasive approach may not be in the best interest of the patient. It may reinforce the belief that the pain has an organic basis and initiate invalidism in a patient without evidence of ascertainable organic disease. The impact of invasive investigations in a patient population with a high prevalence of psychiatric morbidity and hypochondriacal traits is difficult to estimate, but a proportion

Table 18.1 Hyperventilation-provocation test

1 The patient should be seated and informed that she is going to be subjected to a breathing test. The patient should not be told in advance of the possible consequences of the test

2 The doctor should show the rate and depth he requires the patient to breathe (40 breaths/minute is usual)

3 The patient should be encouraged to describe the sensations he experiences during hyperventilation. The test should continue for 3 minutes, and the aim is to produce hypocapnia of 14–20 mmHg. Ideally this should be checked on a mass spectrometer. If hypocapnia is not produced, the test is inadequate

4 Replication of at least some of the symptoms should have occurred by 3 minutes. If coexisting ischaemic heart disease is suspected in patients with angina-like chest pain, the test should be carried out along with ECG monitoring

5 Refrain from asking leading or closed questions about the symptoms produced. It is better if the patient can make the connection spontaneously before asking if the symptoms are familiar

6 If the test produces symptoms the patient should be encouraged to breathe into a paper bag to show how they can be controlled

become chronic invalids.[27] Four months after angiography 20 per cent of our patients still believed they had heart disease although they had very clearly been shown they were normal and told to lead normal lives.[8]

After the angiogram the history should be retaken. If there is a suggestion of oesophageal disease it should be investigated. All other patients should be told they have a favourable prognosis and encouraged to lead a normal life without restrictions. Cardiac medication should be withdrawn thereby reinforcing the normality. Patients should be reviewed by their family doctor two to three months after angiography to make certain they have returned to a healthy level of activity without complaints. They should not be given a cardiac appointment, ie, they should be discharged after the angiogram (the appointment may reinforce doubts). If the problem continues at two to three months the family doctor should refer for psychiatric assessment in a general hospital. Only at the point of discovering no psychological factors (very unlikely) should invasive procedures be undertaken by a cardiologist. A trial of calcium antagonists would seem to be more in the patient's best interest. This strategy is summarized in Figure 18.2, which also serves as practical points.

19
Ventricular arrhythmias in chronic coronary artery disease

This chapter principally concerns the need for and indications for antiarrhythmic therapy in the ambulant patient who may well have arrhythmias that are symptomatic (palpitations, syncope, heart failure) or have arrhythmias detected by chance at physical examination or on routine ECG.

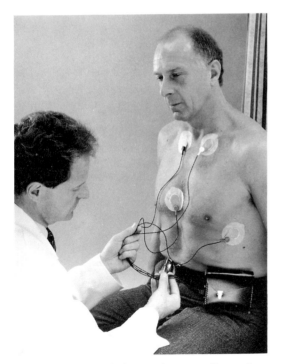

Figure 19.1 Ambulatory electrocardiography. Small portable cassette recorder enabling easy mobility.

INCIDENCE

Ventricular arrhythmias are common. If ambulatory ECG recordings (see Figure 19.1) are taken, ventricular extrasystoles will be recorded in up to 90 per cent of patients with known coronary artery disease (CAD) but ventricular tachycardia (three or more ventricular extrasystoles consecutively) in less than 5 per cent.[1,2] Ventricular extrasystoles are less likely to be detected by exercise electrocardiography, occurring in 50 per cent with a similar 5 per cent risk of ventricular tachycardia.[3]

Implications

The problem with ventricular arrhythmias is the lack of a clear relationship between them and mortality (sudden death). As has been discussed before (see page 112) the mortality appears to be related to left ventricular dysfunction with which ventricular arrhythmias are associated. Thus they may be a marker of mortality rather than the cause.

Trying to clarify subsets at risk, Lown evolved his famous classification based on the assumption that the more severe the arrhythmia the greater the risk of sudden death (see Table 19.1),[4] with grades 4 and 5 imparting substantially increased risks of sudden death.

Unfortunately even taking this into account, no consistent benefit has been recorded from intervention and, furthermore, sudden death caused by ventricular fibrillation may occur without any warning arrhythmias.[5] It is true to say, however, that most people with grade 4 and 5 arrhythmias are symptomatic, so a decision to treat is made easier.

TYPES OF ARRHYTHMIAS

Asymptomatic ventricular arrhythmias

There is no evidence that treatment is worthwhile for ventricular extrasystoles. Patients who have ventricular tachycardia or have survived recurrent fibrillation should receive therapy since there is evidence suggesting benefit in one study, although the suppression of the arrhythmia may simply be a way of identifying a person who will do well anyway. It is conceivable that the ventricular arrhythmia is a marker of risk and its suppression a marker of survival rather than cause and benefit from therapy (see Figure 19.2). Table 19.2 summarizes the arguments for and against drug intervention. The basis of good management, however, begins with assessment of heart failure and treatment, correction of electrolyte disturbance and avoidance of any agent known to induce arrhythmias.

Symptomatic ventricular arrhythmias

When extrasystoles are frequent and easily perceived by the patient they should be suppressed in order to maintain quality of life. Again the first step is to remove any precipitating cause. Always check for a history of stress and try to identify a means of reducing it. Caffeine in tea, coffee and Coca-Cola may be a problem and alcohol can be an irritant too. Smoking is bad generally but may contribute to symptomatic arrhythmias as may some medications involved in the therapy of asthma or depression. If the arrhythmia persists a therapeutic option should take into account any other background complaint, eg, beta-blockade if there is angina. Other drug therapy involves specific antiarrhythmic agents.

CLASSIFICATION OF ANTIARRHYTHMIC DRUGS

This group of drugs causes many side-effects, affecting the gastrointestinal tract and central nervous system in particular. Many are negatively inotropic and can cause heart failure and hypotension and some, by virtue of their actions on the conducting system, can replace one problem with another by turning ventricular arrhythmias into heart block.

Table 19.1 Lown's grading system for ventricular arrhythmias

Grade	Definition
0	No extrasystoles
1	< 30 in 1 hour
2	> 30 in 1 hour
3	Multifocal extrasystoles
4a	Couplets/pairs, ie, 2 consecutive extrasystoles
4b	3 or more consecutive extrasystoles (ventricular tachycardia)
5	R-on-T extrasystoles

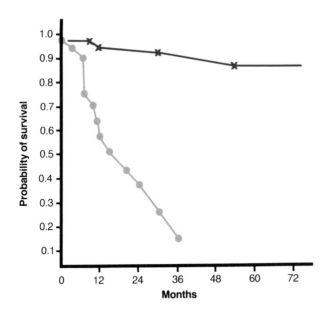

Figure 19.2 Probability of sudden death related to control (X) or not(●) of ventricular extrasystoles in 123 patients with ventricular tachycardia or fibrillation.

Table 19.2 Asymptomatic ventricular arrhythmias – decision to treat

For	Against
1 The rhythms are associated with sudden death	Association does not mean cause
2 Drugs used individually are highly effective	Consistent suppression is not frequently seen, ie, it is not sustained
3 Ventricular fibrillation can be prevented	Only one study shows this.[6] Many more do not[5]
4 The drugs act to suppress unwanted beats	Occasionally they can be 'proarrhythmic' and worsen the situation[7]

Clinical approach

This is the most useful way of thinking about drugs and translating their mode and site of action into clinical use[8] (see Table 19.3). By noting a site of action, a range of effectiveness follows, eg, amiodarone and flecainide deal with supraventricular and ventricular arrhythmias, while mexiletine affects only ventricular arrhythmias.

Electrophysiological classification

This stems from the work of Vaughan-Williams,[9] resulting from studying the electrophysiological action at cellular level. This is really a research classification of limited clinical use (see Table 19.4). The classification can be summarized as follows:

Class I These drugs restrict sodium movement across the cell membrane, reducing the rate of rise of the action poten-

Site	Drug
Sinus node	Beta-blockers, digoxin, verapamil, procainamide, disopyramide, amiodarone, quinidine
Atrioventricular node	Digoxin, verapamil, beta-blockers (? diltiazem) flecainide
Anomalous pathway (eg, Wolff-Parkinson-White syndrome)	Disopyramide, amiodarone, procainamide, quinidine, flecainide
Ventricles	Lignocaine, disopyramide, tocainide, mexiletine, phenytoin, procainamide, quinidine, amiodarone, flecainide

Table 19.3   Sites of action of antiarrhythmic drugs

	I	II	III	IV
A	Quinidine	Beta-blockers	Amiodarone	Verapamil
	Procainamide	Bretylium	Sotalol	Diltiazem
	Disopyramide		Bretylium	
B	Lignocaine			
	Mexiletine			
	Tocainide			
	Phenytoin			
C	Flecainide			

Table 19.4   Classification based on electrophysiology (Vaughan-Williams)

tial (see Figure 19.3). IA drugs lengthen, IB shorten and IC do not affect the duration of the action potential. Thus IB drugs work at ventricular level whereas IA and IC can affect the atria and the ventricle.

Class II These interfere with the sympathetic nervous system and reduce the potential for arrhythmias secondary to raised catecholamines.

Class III These extend the duration of the action potential, thereby prolonging the effective refractory period.

Class IV These inhibit the transport of calcium across the cell membrane which follows the inward movement of sodium, thus depressing phase 2 and 3 of the action potential. The most sensitive area for effect is the sinus and atrioventricular node.

Drugs for ventricular arrhythmias

The limited effectiveness of the agents and the high incidence of side-effects should be emphasized again. At this point it is important to be certain that there is no correctable cause for the arrhythmia. Symptoms are principally being treated and this means the drugs

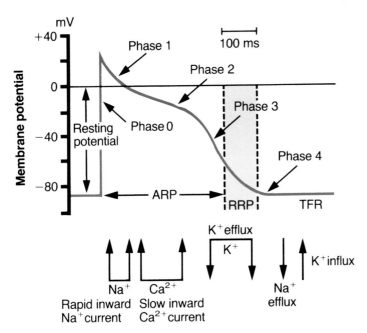

Figure 19.3 Action potential. ARP=Absolute refractory period; RRP=relative refractory period; TFR=time of full recovery.

being used should make the patient feel better. It is better to have one or two extrasystoles that can be tolerated than none at the expense of drug side-effects. The drug doses and adverse effects are summarized in Table 19.5.

A strategy

1   If there is no substantial impairment of ventricular function adminster:

- Beta-blockade as anti-ischaemia
- Flecainide
- Amiodarone
- Mexiletine.

2   If there is clinical heart failure administer:

- Amiodarone
- Other drugs with very great care.

3   Resistant and dangerous arrhythmias— try combinations (in hospital) eg, amiodarone plus flecainide.

Monitoring effects

If the patient feels better then that is the index for success for symptomatic ventricular extrasystoles. If the indication for therapy was symptomatic or asymptomatic ventricular tachycardia, 24-hour ECG recordings should be used to assess effectiveness.[6] They may also identify any proarrhythmic effects also.[7] Proarrhythmic refers to the genesis of an arrhythmia by drugs. This often occurs when the QT is prolonged and one of the most frequently seen is torsade de pointes ventricular tachycardia (see page 116). It does not seem logical to treat an asymptomatic arrhythmia without monitoring the effect — how can we know if the intervention is effective?

Plasma concentrations are not necessary if an objective benefit from therapy can be seen but they may be very useful to judge compliance and clear up any confusion regarding symptoms of toxicity.

OTHER OPTIONS

Intracardiac electrophysiological testing

This usually involves stopping all medication and trying to induce the arrhythmia in patients who have had ventricular tachycardia or fibrillation.[10,11] Drugs can then be used to prevent it occurring and their effectiveness tested. Clearly this is invasive, expensive and requires sophisticated technology. Side-effects of drug treatment are frequent and suppression not complete, but in those with recurrent problems not responding to conventional attempts at suppression it is claimed that in two-thirds a regime can be found.

This procedure should be used when there is failure to control an arrhythmia with amiodarone in combination with another agent, eg, flecainide.

Cardiac surgery

Bypass surgery may prevent recurrent arrhythmias but does not influence overall survival.[12] Resection of a left ventricular aneurysm can be effective on its own[13] but current emphasis is on mapping techniques which identify what is believed to be the exact source of the arrhythmias.[14,15] Resection or cryoablation of that area follows.[16] This approach is for patients refractory to drug therapy who are not suitable for bypass surgery which may be indicated for other reasons, eg, angina.

Implantable defibrillators

These are now becoming available for patients with recurrent arrhythmias who fail to respond to other therapy. Their safety and reliability are unknown at present but if all else has failed and a specialist centre is available they provide yet another option.[17]

Drug (generic name)	Dosage	Therapeutic range	Adverse effects	Comment
Lignocaine	100 mg iv bolus 50 mg at 5 minutes if needed 1–4 mg/minute infusion	1.5–5.0 mg/l	More likely in cardiac failure + liver disease, Nausea, vomiting, paraesthesiae, twitching, convulsions	First choice acute infarct. Low K$^+$ impairs effect
Mexiletine	Oral 200–300 mg tds. Perlongets 360 mg bid iv, 100–250 mg 5–10 minutes, 250 mg then over 1 hour, 250 mg over 2 hours, then 0.5–1.0 mg/minute	0.75–2.0 mg/l	Common: nausea, vomiting, confusion, ataxia, tremor, bradycardia	Prolongets less side-effects
Tocainide	Oral 400 mg tds or 600 mg bid iv 750 mg over 15 minutes	6–12 mg/l	Renal impairment worsens. Anorexia, nausea, vomiting, constipation. Rashes. CNS as mexiletine. Blood dyscrasias.	Adverse profile worrying.
Disopyramide	iv 1.5–2.0 mg/kg to 150 mg over 5–10 minutes, 20–30 mg/h to 800 mg. Oral 300–800 mg daily (tds). Slow release 300 mg bid	2–5 mg/l	Hypotension and failure iv. Oral — dry mouth, blurred vision, urine retention. QT prolongation. Sinus node depression. Glaucoma	Renal excretion Avoid iv
Flecainide	iv 2 mg/kg over 10–20 minutes. Oral 100–200 mg bid	200–1000 ng/ml	Visual disturbance, lightheaded. Prolongs QT: proarrhythmic. Negatively inotropic + pacing threshhold increased	Potent, effective drug > 90 per cent effective. Beware cardiac failures
Amiodarone	3.5 mg/kg iv 5 minute (central line) Oral 200 mg tds 1 week then 100 or 200 mg daily	unknown	Corneal deposits. Photosensitivity (30 per cent). Thyroid disturbance (2–3 per cent). Nausea, alopecia, blue skin, tremor, nightmares. Pulmonary fibrosis, neuropathy, myopathy. QT prolonged	Drug interactions (digoxin, warfarin). Very effective drug, safe in heart failure
Quinidine	Kinidin durules 500 mg bid	2.0–5 mg/l	Gastrointestinal frequent. Tinnitus, deafness. Hypotension. Raises digoxin concentrations. QT prolonged. Cinchonism fever, purpura, thrombocytopenia.	Best reserved for atrial fibrillation *with* digoxin
Procainamide	iv 100 mg/minute to 1 g, then 2–6 mg/minute Oral — durules 1.0–1.5 g 8 hourly	4.0–10 mg/l	Gastrointestinal frequent. Hypotension. SLE myopathy. Slow acetylators lower doses. QT prolonged. Heart block	Good iv if lignocaine not effective.

Notes
1. All drugs are toxic.
2. Intravenous lignocaine is simple and effective but beware of different ampoule concentrations.
3. If lignocaine ineffective try procainamide then amiodarone. If no effect use bretylium 5 mg/kg.
4. Oral therapy – consider beta-blockade for ischaemia.
5. Most effective is flecainide but not recommended in heart failure.
6. Amiodarone in heart failure and when other drugs fail or the problem is a mixture of supraventricular and ventricular arrhythmias.
7. When faced with an intravenous drug and you cannot remember the dose never use more than one ampoule without double-checking the dosage.

Table 19.5 Drugs for ventricular arrhythmias

PRACTICAL POINTS

- Ventricular extrasystoles that are asymptomatic can be ignored.

- If treatment is contemplated a non-drug approach should the the first option.

- Asymptomatic ventricular tachycardia and symptomatic arrhythmias merit therapy.

- Most agents have side-effects and many are negatively inotropic.

- 24-hour ECG monitoring is not necessary unless ventricular tachycardia is being suppressed.

- Resistant cases should be referred to specialist centres for mapping and surgery.

Non-cardiac surgery in patients with ischaemic heart disease

Surgery and anaesthesia pose stresses for the cardiovascular system which may precipitate myocardial infarction. The mechanisms involve hypovolaemia after haemorrhage leading to hypotension and ischaemia, hypoxia during ventilation, and excess of catecholamines increasing heart rate and oxygen demand in the presence of decreased supply and the absence of warning pain.

PREVIOUS INFARCTION

The incidence of operative infarction is 6.6 per cent in those which previous events compared with 0.66 per cent for those without previous infarction.[1] The mortalities are strikingly different at 70 per cent and 26.5 per cent, respectively. If the operation is carried out within six months the reported incidence is 50 per cent compared with 1 per cent at three years.[2,3] The Mayo clinic reported similar findings with a 6.6 per cent operative infarct, 37 per cent infarct rate if the operation was inside three months of the infarct, 16 per cent after three months and 4.5 per cent after six months.[4,5]

None of these studies include risk stratification by early postinfarction exercise testing; thus they are to some extent out of date. It seems sensible to advise a six-month delay for non-life-threatening conditions, eg, hernias. If an early exercise test is negative for additional ischaemia, this provides reassurance. If an early exercise test is abnormal, angiography should be done and the patient treated with beta-blockade. The patient may well need cardiac surgery to enable non-cardiac surgery to proceed at an acceptable risk. If the surgery is essential to save life then the risks should be explained to the patient.

ANGINA PECTORIS

The risks are the same as for the first six months after infarction. The risks are greater with surgery of the great vessels, thorax or upper abdomen.[5] Mortality increases with age, being 10 per cent at fifty to fifty-nine, 15 per cent at sixty to sixty-nine and 25 per cent at over seventy years of age, approximately double those without coronary artery disease.[6]

Those who have mild angina and a normal or minimally changed exercise ECG are better surgical risks than those with moderate to severe angina and a positive ischaemic ECG.[7]

CARDIAC FAILURE

The surgical mortality ranges from 4–10 per cent in mild failure to 10–20 per cent with moderate failure and 30–70 per cent with severe heart failure.[8] The decision must be taken on the severity of the condition, eg, hernias in patients with severe failure should be managed with a truss. Bleeding ulcers are always a high risk but, if necessary, surgery can be chanced.

Recommendations

1 Delay elective surgery for six months after infarction.

2 Establish risk status as routine with

exercise testing. Define any cardiac problem if possible.

3 Within six months of infarction or in the presence of severe angina or heart failure, an operation depends entirely on its life-threatening implications.

4 For those who are at high risk (age over seventy, previous infarct) but who are disabled by the pain of their illness (eg, osteoarthritis of the hip) it is reasonable to allow surgery to go ahead providing all parties understand the risk. In this group, angiography with a view to angioplasty or surgery may allow elective non-cardiac surgery to proceed safely after appropriate cardiac intervention.

5 Post-operative cardiac care unit supervision is desirable.

6 A cardiac opinion is recommended for all cases.

PREOPERATIVE CARE

Angina
A long acting beta-blocker (eg, atenolol 100 mg) 6 hours before surgery will give protection for 24 hours. Intravenous nitrates can be started before and maintained for 24–48 hours postoperation.

Heart failure
Medication should continue up to 6 hours before surgery. More severe cases should be monitored with pulmonary artery and arterial lines along with urinary catheters. Intravenous diuretics, inotropes and vasodilators may be necessary.

Endocarditis prophylaxis
This is needed only for associated or independent valvar pathology.

21
Case histories

1 Mrs B aged forty-seven presented with rest pain. The ECG showed pronounced anterior lateral ST depression (see Figure 21.1) but no evidence of acute infarction. Cardiac enzymes did not rise. She was managed conventionally with intravenous nitrates and aspirin but persistence of symptoms required therapy with beta-blockade and calcium antagonists to establish control. After being stabilized (see Figure 21.2) adopting our routine policy, she was transferred from the district hospital to King's College Hospital for angiography. The ECG suggested a left main stem lesion.

Figure 21.3 shows the alarming nature of her problem with a critical mainstem lesion. She was continued on bed rest, intravenous nitrates and subcutaneous heparin. Elective bypass surgery was a total success.

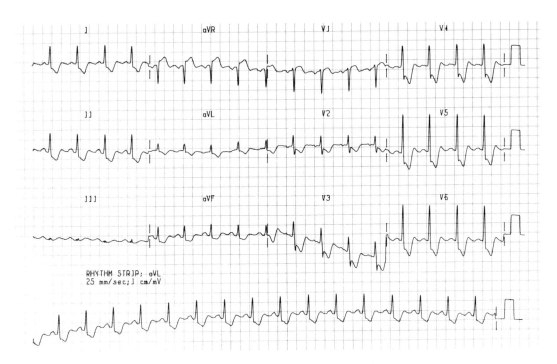

Figure 21.1 Dramatic anterolateral ST depression of unstable angina.

Comment

Unstable angina is a dangerous condition and when the facilities are available to establish risk we can identify individuals whose life depends on surgical intervention. In this case the ECG almost 'shouted' a warning.

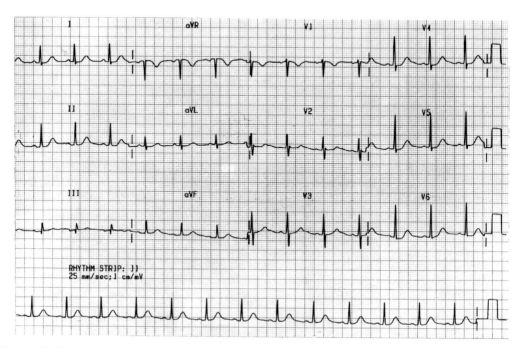

Figure 21.2 Resolution of ECG changes after medical therapy. A normal ECG does not rule out the existence of significant CAD.

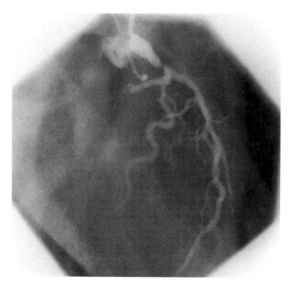

Figure 21.3 Case 1: Critical left main stem lesion.

2 Mr V aged forty years gave a two-month history of tight chest pain waking him early in the morning at 5 am. He was a heavy smoker. He had no effort pain. One month previously he had presented to casualty after a particularly severe pain but the ECG was normal and he was sent home.

The symptoms continued and again a severe pain caused presentation to casualty. This time the ECG during pain showed ST elevation (see Figure 21.4) and he was admitted. This is a typical case of Prinzmetal's angina. He was stabilized on intravenous then oral nitrates combined with diltiazem. In view of his smoking the likely diagnosis was spasm on a fixed obstructive lesion. Routine angiography showed a 99 per cent proximal left anterior descending (LAD) lesion and 70 per cent long atheromatous right coronary lesion (see Figure 21.5).

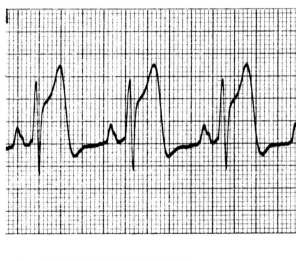

Figure 21.4 Case 2: ST elevation during pain.

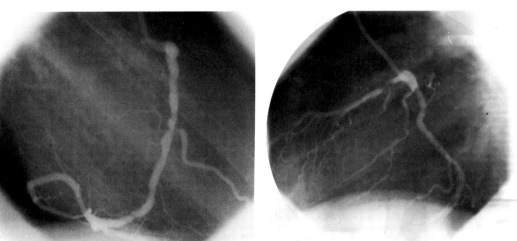

Figure 21.5 Prinzmetal's angina. Angiogram shows significant LAD stenosis (right) and right coronary atheroma (left).

He was referred for internal mammary artery grafting and calcium antagonists were continued after the operation.

Comment

Failure to take a proper history and being blinkered by the ECG is highlighted in this case when he was sent home. The subsequent management involved antispasm agents, defining the anatomy and elective surgery. Spasm can recur after operation but it cannot be predicted in whom. Therapy should be continued therefore, even though surgery is anatomically successful.

3 Mr M aged thirty-six sustained an inferior infarct. It was uncomplicated, but in view of his age and heavy smoking routine angiography was carried out. This identified a 90 per cent proximal LAD lesion and a blocked right coronary artery.

He was referred for surgery on prognostic grounds but because of financial constraints this was delayed for three months. During this time he sustained a large anterior infarct and died from cardiac failure.

Comment

If we identify risks we must be able to implement the necessary treatment.

4 Mr L had a familial hypercholesterolaemia managed by diet and cholestyramine. He was followed at yearly intervals and remained asymptomatic. At each visit he had a maximal exercise test. After five normal years when aged thirty-seven the test became abnormal. In view of the change he was referred for angiography. This identified critical three vessel coronary artery disease and he underwent successful bypass surgery. He continues annual stress tests which are now normal.

Comment

Familial hypercholesterolaemia represents a high risk for coronary disease. Annual exer-

198

cise testing may be a way of identifying the development of significant coronary disease before a complication occurs.

5 Mr N sustained an acute inferior infarction at age forty-six years. He developed heart block and was temporarily paced. Progress was satisfactory until the third day when he had a cardiac arrest. The main feature of the arrest was electromechanical dissociation, ie, he had electrical (paced) complexes but no cardiac output. It was decided he had either had a massive pulmonary embolus, infarct extension, or had ruptured giving him tamponade. As there was nothing to lose a needle was advanced to the pericardium, blood was aspirated and immediately his output returned. A catheter was passed into the pericardium and, being continuously aspirated, he was taken to theatre.

The surgeon found a hole in the right ventricle. The infarct had extended to the area where the pacemaker wire was positioned and it had perforated. The story has a happy ending with us drinking champagne with the patient the next day—his wedding anniversary.

Comment

When all else is lost at resuscitation and complexes occur with no output, tamponade should be excluded.

6 A consultant physician of sixty years of age sustained an acute inferior infarct in the Middle East. He collapsed suddenly on the second day and a murmur was heard. In cardiogenic shock, he was airlifted to King's College Hospital where a ruptured ventricular septal defect (VSD) was immediately identified. Emergency angiography showed single vessel disease with a large shunt. A balloon pump was inserted percutaneously and he was stabilized. Because the hole was close to the aortic valve the surgeon wished to delay until fibrosis gave his sutures chance to hold.

He was managed for three weeks on the balloon pump, occasionally using inotropes. Pericarditis-induced atrial fibrillation and septicaemia were treated and he subsequently underwent successful surgery. It was complicated by transient weakness of the left leg. At eighteen months he has a normal exercise ECG and is playing golf and planning to ski.

Comment
Cardiogenic shock is reversible if the problem is a mechanical defect. Usually surgery is best done early but in this case, because of the location of the VSD, a successful delayed procedure was undertaken.

7   Mrs B aged forty-eight sustained an anterior subendocardial infarct (see Figure 21.6). She underwent routine angiography one week later which identified a 90 per cent stenosis in the LAD. She proceeded to angiop-

lasty which was totally successful (see Figure 21.7). At follow-up for three years repeat angiography confirms the improvement.

Comment
Subendocardial infarction has a high rate of cardiac events in the subsequent year. In this case a critical lesion was identified and successfully treated with angioplasty.

8   Mrs O aged fifty-two developed unstable angina and continued to have chest pain on medical therapy. Angiography showed a critical LAD lesion. Angioplasty was successfully carried out. However, 10 minutes later the patient collapsed, the blood pressure fell to 40 mmHg and electromechanical dissociation occurred. Full resuscitation was started. Angiography revealed an occluded vessel. This was reopened by angioplasty and remained open. Output, however, did not

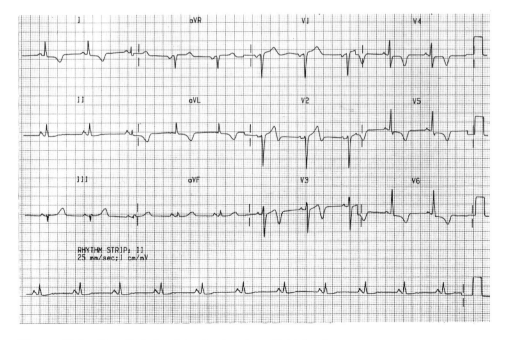

Figure 21.6   Case 7: Anterolateral subendocardial infarct.

improve. A balloon pump was inserted. No infarct was demonstrated. After 2 hours of resuscitation the patient died. At post-mortem examination the artery was patent; there was no dissection or evidence of infarction.

Comment

It is still not known what happened. Cases like this reinforce the need for carefully controlled studies to establish the place of angioplasty.

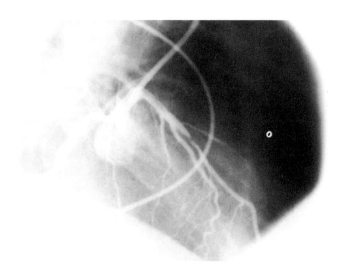

Figure   21.7 Angiogram showing LAD lesion before (top) and after successful angioplasty (bottom).

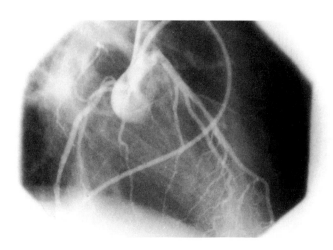

Appendix 1

King's College Hospital cardiac care guide

It is hoped that the following brief outline will help junior medical staff in the management of myocardial infarction and its complications. There is a 24-hour seven day cardiac service; use it if there are problems. We would appreciate any discussion. The author and publishers would be happy for this guide to be reproduced with or without amendments.

SELECTION OF PATIENTS FOR ADMISSION TO THE CARDIAC CARE UNIT

- Those who are suspected of having had a myocardial infarct less than 10 hours previously
- Those with arrhythmias, shock or other major complications
- Those who are likely candidates for an infarct within a number of days, ie, patients with unstable angina (intermediate coronary syndrome)
- Specific cardiotoxic drug overdoses
- The coronary unit is *not* an overflow unit nor is it a general medical intensive care
- Age less than seventy-five years but use discretion.

Early admission important

Patients should be detained in the casualty department only as long as is necessary to make the diagnosis, relieve pain, insert an intravenous line and treat any serious arrhythmias.

Investigations

- Portable chest x-ray to assess lung fields as soon as possible after arrival at cardiac care unit (casualty only if unavoidable delay)
- Creatine phosphokinase (CPK) on day of admission
- CPK daily for first two days
- Daily ECG for first two days (and ECGs during pain)
- Daily chest x-ray in acute coronary wing.

GENERAL THERAPY

Analgesia

If the pain is severe diamorphine 5 mg by slow intravenous injection followed by a further 2.5 mg at 10 minutes if severe pain persists. (NB Care should be taken if patient has chronic respiratory failure.) Give antiemetic, eg, cyclizine 50 mg iv. This is preferable to metoclopramide because of central mode of action.

Oxygen

Need not be given routinely. Give in presence of cardiac failure, shock, cyanosis or prolonged pain. Use oxygenaire safety mask at 8 l/min or medium concentration (MC) mask at

4 1/min unless there is evidence of chronic lung disease when blood gas analysis will be necessary for assessment of the patient both prior to and during oxygen therapy. (Safe dose usually 25 per cent.)

Posture

Semirecumbent or, if distressed, in whatever position is comfortable.

Physiotherapy

Encourage leg movement throughout admission in all patients.

Sedation

If necessary; diazepam 2–10 mg tds (care if patient has chronic lung disease).

Intravenous line

'Venflon' iv cannula. Preferably not cubital fossa vein.

Nitrates

For persisting pain use sublingual GTN or spray. If pain continues establish isosorbide dinitrate infusion (2 mg/hour) increasing at 30 minute intervals if pain persists. Monitor blood pressure carefully to keep SBP > 90 mmHg. If stable, mononitrate 20 mg bid increasing to 40 mg bid can be started.

Anticoagulant therapy

Heparin 5000 units subcutaneously 8 hourly until patient is fully mobilized.

Diet

Light.

Temperature

Maintain unit 70°F (20°C).

Bowels

If stay is longer than 48 hours use lactulose. Commode.

Left ventricular failure (orthopnoea, III sound, pulsus alternans, basal crackles, chest x-ray changes)

- Diamorphine 5 mg by slow intravenous injection (unless recently given for its analgesic effect). [Remember chronic obstructive airways disease (COAD).]
- Sit the patient up
- Oxygen—high concentration (except COAD)
- Frusemide 40–80 mg iv followed by intravenous or oral therapy. Repeat if necessary (K^+). Remember elderly male prostrate glands (use 20 mg iv)
- Aminophylline 250–500 mg by intravenous infusion given *over at least 10 minutes* if wheezing is a major component
- Nitrate infusion as above
- Digitalize if ventricular rate persistently greater than 100 beats/minute after diuretic therapy (or correct underlying arrhythmia)
- Nitroprusside for afterload reduction for left ventricular failure if failing to respond to the above—maintain SBP > 90 mmHg
- Artificial ventilation if exhausted
- Peritoneal dialysis ⎫ in
- Venesection 1 litre ⎭ desperation

Cardiogenic shock (pallor, blood pressure less than 90 mmHg systolic, cold clammy extremities, oliguria)

- Posture—the position found most comfortable by the patient
- Relieve pain—diamorphine
- Treatment of arrhythmias —urgent; treat with dc shock and do not use cardiac suppressants
- Oxygen therapy—high inspiratory concentration
- Correction of acidosis = check pH. Use 8.4 per cent $NaHCO_3$
- Insert urinary catheter
- Thrombolysis and/or angioplasty if inside 6 hours (act quickly).

If no response to treatment within half an hour: call cardiac registrar

Swan-Ganz catheter (or central venous pressure line). If:

1 Near normal or even low right atrial pressure < 5 mm or pulmonary atrial pressure (rare) < 15 mmHg mean. Infusion of 500 ml 5 per cent dextrose over 30 minutes. If improvement without dangerous increase in right atrial pressure or pulmonary artery diastolic pressure dextran infusion.
2 Right atrial pressure greater than 10 cm of water (usual case). Increase cardiac output with dopamine 5 µg/kg per minute and dobutamine 5 µg/kg per minute to 25 µg/minute (or isoprenaline 1–2 µg/minute increased up to 5 µg/minute), provided favourable response occurs without excessive tachycardia. Or salbutamol 7–25 µg/minute. Frusemide 40 mg up to 500 mg iv as required.

If no response, consider:

1 Methylprednisolone 30 mg/kg iv bolus given over 10 minutes, and repeat once or twice in the next 24 hours only. Central venous pressure must be over 10 cm.
2 Intra-aortic balloon. Consider balloon early, age less than sixty-five years and infarct less than 4 hours. Dopamine or salbutamol + inotropic support must be given prior to or with balloon. If less than 4 hours since infarct plan coronary angiograms with a view to surgery or thrombolysis or angioplasty. Balloon for later shock only delays death and makes it more miserable.

SUPRAVENTRICULAR TACHYCARDIA

Try carotid sinus massage.

If no response practolol 5 mg every 5 minutes to maximum 25 mg iv or:

1 Atenolol 1–5 mg iv over 5 minutes to a maximum dose of 10 mg or rapid digitilization providing that no previous digitalis preparations have been used.
2 If no response or if severe and associated with heart failure, hypotension or recurrence of chest pain—dc shock (100 joules, then increase).
3 Consider verapamil 5–10 mg iv over 30 seconds as alternative to practolol. It is *not advisable* in patients previously digitalized or given beta-blockers because of the risk of inducing asystole. Remember it is negatively intropic. It is highly effective.
4 Amiodarone 300 mg iv over 20 minutes to one hour in 5 per cent dextrose.

ATRIAL FIBRILLATION AND ATRIAL FLUTTER

May be transient and not associated with haemodynamic deterioration. If more prolonged with rapid ventricular rate—digitalize, beta-block or give verapamil. Check for pericarditis first (re steroids or indomethacin) and assess for failure. If associated with haemodynamic deterioration—dc shock (dc shock after previous digitalis therapy should be initially of low energy—20–50 joules).

DIGITALIZATION

Emergency digitalization (provided patient has not had digitalis during the previous six weeks). In cases with a rapid ventricular rate (more than 100 beats/minute) and failure or fibrillation.

Digoxin 0.5 mg slowly intravenously, followed after 60 minutes by a further 0.25 mg iv, then by oral digitalization schedule. Omit 0.25 mg dose if patient older than seventy or urea greater than twice normal.

Routine oral digitalization

Day 1—0.5 mg tds
Day 2—0.25 mg bd
Day 3 and subsequently—0.25 mg om

If blood urea more than 8 mmol (48 mg/100 ml) halve all maintenance doses. If in doubt measure digoxin level.

VENTRICULAR ECTOPICS

Indications for treatment

Increasing in number (more than six/minute).
Consecutive ectopics (salvoes or couplets).
Multifocal.

R-on-T.
Post ventricular fibrillation for 24 hours.

Treatment

With bradycardia atropine 0.3–1.2 mg iv.

Without bradycardia lignocaine 100 mg iv over 2 minutes followed by further 50 mg iv if no response. If liver function impaired halve doses.

If response occurs, continue with lignocaine 4 mg/minute for 1 hour then 2 mg/minute increasing to 2–4 mg/minute in 5 per cent dextrose as necessary. (Overdosage may cause fits, confusion, hypotension, increasing heart failure, and coma and is more likely in the presence of liver disease or low cardiac output states.)

If no response to lignocaine try procainamide 50–100 mg by slow (5 minutes) intravenous injection increasing to effect or 1 g or amiodarone 300 mg iv.

Oral therapy if required

1 Mexiletine 200 mg tds, disopyramide 100 mg tds–200 mg tds, flecainide 100–200 mg bid, amiodarone 400 mg tds, two days 200 mg tds, five days then 200 mg daily. Only amiodarone if in failure
2 Procainamide durules 1.5 g tds.
3 Beta-blockade.

VENTRICULAR TACHYCARDIA

Runs of three or more successive ventricular extrasystoles.

Treatment

Lignocaine 100 mg iv.

Correct acidosis if tachycardia has been prolonged with sodium bicarbonate 8.4 per cent.

If no response dc shock starting with 100 joules and increasing by 50 to 100 joule steps if necessary.

When arrhythmia has been corrected to sinus rhythm continue with lignocaine 2–4 mg/minute for at least 24 hours.

If recurrent tachycardias are a problem consider oral therapy as above. Resistant cases may respond acutely to overdrive pacing or intravenous amiodarone.

VENTRICULAR FIBRILLATION

Direct current shock 200 joules increasing to 400 joules.

Ventilate. External cardiac massage.

Correct acidosis with 50 mmol/l (50 mEq/l) bicarbonate (if necessary monitor response). This recommendation may change in the near future.

If ventricular fibrillation persists try lignocaine 50–100 mg iv and if this fails procainamide 50–100 mg iv repeating the dc shocks then consider bretylium 500 mg iv and/or amiodarone 300 mg iv.

SINUS BRADYCARDIA

Indications for treatment

Heart rate less than 60/minute *plus* hypotension or frequent ventricular ectopics.

Heart rate less than 45 beats/minute *per se* (but judge individual cases).

Treatment

Intravenous atropine aliquots of 0.3 mg (usually to a total of 0.6–1.2 mg but rarely up to 2.7 mg). May need repeat depending on rate.

(There is a risk of a tachycardia occurring during treatment with atropine, so begin with small doses). If no response—atrial pacing.

COMPLETE HEART BLOCK

Consult with cardiac unit resident about pacing as soon as second (Mobitz II) or third degree block occurs.

Treat in emergency with intravenous isoprenaline infusion (1–4 µg/minute). If no response try atropine 0.6 mg aliquots intravenously to maximum of 2.4 mg. This is purely to get the patient to pacing theatre.

PACING

Indications for insertion of a pacemaker

Sinus bradycardia unresponsive to atropine and associated with hypotension and/or cardiac failure.

Heart block of second (Mobitz II) and third degree. Mobitz I if hypotension or brady unresponsive to atropine.

Asystole. This is probably impractical in the vast majority of cases in our present situation. The newer external pacemakers may be used here.

Bundle branch block. Pacing is indicated here when left axis deviation is associated with right bundle branch block, ie, bifascicular block or where there is alternating right and left bundle branch block *and the patient is symptomatic* (syncope).

Overdrive for ventricular arrhythmias.

Asystole

- A sharp blow to the chest
- External chest compression and artificial respiration
- Sodium bicarbonate (as for ventricular fibrillation). Under review
- Adrenaline 2 ml of 1:1000 or 10 cc 1:10 000—repeat as necessary

- Isoprenaline infusion 5–40 µg/minute using massive doses which must be discontinued as soon as possible
- Defibrillate when ventricular fibrillation occurs
- If no intravenous line give endotracheal or intracardiac injections.

Unstable angina

Rapid increasing chest pain, pain at rest, new or severe pain. No ECG or CPK changes. *ECG may well be normal.*

1 Diamorphine + cyclizine as above + aspirin 300 mg daily.
2 Sublingual and intravenous nitrates (isosorbide 2–4 mg/hour or higher). Keep SBP > 90 mmHg.
3 Oral mononitrates (20–40 mg bid) + beta-blockade (atenolol 50–100 mg om).
4 Calcium antagonists if blockade contraindicated, ie, diltiazem 60–120 mg tds or verapamil 40–120 mg tds. Do not use nifedipine without beta-blockade. If used add to beta-blockade 5 mg tds–40 mg bid.
5 Balloon pump—do not procrastinate—call cardiac registrar or surgical registrar.
6 Angiography and surgery.

All cases of unstable angina should be started on intravenous and oral nitrates as soon as possible.

Pericarditis

Can occur in all cases but suspect with atrial tachyarrhythmias.

1 Aspirin 300–600 mg 6 hours. Check peptic ulcer history
2 Indomethacin 25 mg tds Check peptic ulcer history
3 Steroids hydrocortisone 100 mg iv 6 hourly if persistent or severe. Check peptic ulcer history

Thrombolysis

This is a rapidly changing area as newer preparations become available, so check with cardiac team immediately.

Streptokinase

- Consider if infarct less than 4 hours and certainly inside 2 hours. Need to act *very* fast.
- Contact cardiac team immediately.
- Regime—1, iv 1.0 million units over 30 minutes. 2, intracoronary 250 000 units slowly.
- Patient selection critical. Risk of arrhythmias during reperfusion significant.
- Give lignocaine 100 mg iv bolus Hydrocortisone to prevent allergic reaction 100 mg iv.
- Recent surgery, severe hypertension, CVA or peptic ulceration are contraindications.

Notes

The cardiac unit is designed to relieve pain, reassure patients and relatives and begin the rehabilitation of patients. It also exits to prevent avoidable death—if in trouble call for help.

Appendix 2

Useful addresses

British Heart Foundation
102 Gloucester Place
London W1H 4DH

Many excellent booklets aimed at the patient

Flora *Cooking with care*
25 North Row
London W1R 2BY

Excellent book on healthy eating (£1.50)

The Health Education Council
78 New Oxford Street
London WC1A 1AH

Pamphlets and information packs on smoking and life style

The Scottish Health Education Group
Woodburn House
Canaan Lane
Edinburgh EH10 4SG

As above

Action on Smoking and Health
5–11 Mortimer Street
London W1N 7RH

As above

Coronary Prevention Group
Central Middlesex Hospital
Acton Lane
London NW10 7NS

As above

Stuart Pharmaceuticals
Stuart House
50 Alderley Road
Wilmslow
Cheshire SK9 1RE

Selection of patient booklets

Laerdal Medical Ltd
Goodmead Road
Orpington
Kent BR6 OHX

Posters on resuscitation

References

Chapter 1

1 Ross R, Glomset JA, 'The pathogenesis of atherosclerosis', *N Engl J Med* (1976) **25:** pp. 369–77, and 420–5.

2 Ross R, 'The pathogenesis of atherosclerosis—an update', *N Engl J Med* (1986) **314:** pp. 488–500.

3 Matthews JD, 'Ischaemic heart disease: possible genetic markers', *Lancet* (1975) **ii:** pp. 681–5.

4 Moncada S, Higgs EA, Vane JR, 'Human arterial and venous tissues generate prostacyclin (prostaglandin X) a potent inhibitor of platelet aggregation', *Lancet* (1977) **i:** pp. 18–20.

5 Mitchell JRA, 'Prostaglandins in vascular disease—a seminal approach', *Br Med J* (1981) **282:** pp. 590–4.

6 Samuelsson B, Hainberg M, Malmsten C, Svensson J, 'The role of prostaglandin endoperoxides and thromboxanes in platelet aggregation', *Adv Prostaglandin Thromboxane Res* (1976) **2:** pp. 237–46.

7 Rutherford RB, Ross R, 'Platelet factors stimulate fibroblasts and smooth muscle cells quiescent in plasma serum to proliferate', *J Cell Biol* (1976) **69:** pp. 196–203.

8 Benditt EP, Benditt JM, 'Evidence for a monoclonal origin of human atherosclerotic plaques', *Proc Natl Acad Sci USA* (1973) **70:** pp. 1753–6.

9 Fulton WFM, 'The pathogenesis of myocardial infarction' in Sleight P, Vann Jones J (eds.), *Scientific foundations cardiology* (Heinemann. London 1983), pp. 213–9.

10 Davies MJ, Fulton WFM, Robertson WB, 'The relation of coronary thrombosis to ischaemic myocardial necrosis', *J Pathol* (1979) **127:** pp. 99–110.

11 Rentrop P, Blanke H, Karseh KR, Kaiser H, Kostering H, Leitz K, 'Selective intracoronary thrombolysis in acute myocardial infarction, *Circulation* (1981) **63:** pp. 307–17.

12 Kennedy J Ward, 'The intracoronary streptokinase treatment of acute myocardial infarction', in Goodwin JF, Yu PN, (eds.), *Progress in cardiology 12.* (Lea and Febiger. Philadelphia 1983), pp. 283–9.

13 Davies MJ, Thomas AC, 'Plaque fissuring—the cause of acute myocardial infarction, sudden ischaemic death and crescendo angina', *Br Heart J* (1985) **53:** pp. 363–73.

14 Smith SH, Geer JC, 'Morphology of saphenous vein—coronary artery bypass grafts', *Arch Pathol Lab Med* (1983) **107:** pp. 13–20.

Chapter 2

1 Tunstall Pedoe H, 'Coronary heart disease' in Miller DL, Farmer RDT (eds.) *Epidemiology of diseases.* (Blackwell. Oxford 1982).

2 Central Statistics Office, *Anual abstract of statistics 1978.* HMSO. London 1982).

3 Office of Population Censuses and Surveys, *Mortality statistics 1980.* HMSO. London 1980.

4 World Health Organization, *Prevention of coronary heart disease.* Technical report series. No 678. WHO. Geneva 1982.

5 Fulton M, 'Regional differences in mortality from ischaemic heart disease and cerebrovascular diseases in Britain', *Br Heart J* (1978) **40:** pp. 563–7.

6 Heller RF, Hayward D, Hobbs MST, 'Decline in rate of death from ischaemic heart disease in the United Kingdom', *Br Med J* (1983) **286:** pp. 260–2.

7   Marmot MG, Rose G, Shipley M, Hamilton PJS, 'Employment grade and coronary heart disease in British civil servants', *J Epidemiol Commun Health* (1978) **32:** pp. 244–9.

8   Clayton DG, Taylor D, Shaper AG, 'Trends in heart disease in England and Wales, 1950–1973', *Health Trends* (1977) **9:** pp. 1–6.

9   Nicholls ES, Jung J, Davies JW, 'Cardiovascular disease mortality in Canada', *Can Med Assoc J* (1981) **125:** pp. 981–92.

10 Salonen JT, Puska P, Kottke TE, Tuomilehto J, Nissinen A, 'Decline in mortality from coronary heart disease in Finland from 1969–1979', *Br Med J* (1983) **286:** pp. 1857–60.

11 Alfredson L, Ahlbom A, 'Increasing incidence and mortality from myocardial infarction in Stockholm country', *Br Med J* (1983) **286:** pp. 1931–3.

12 Epstein FH, Pisaz Z, 'International comparisons in ischaemic heart disease mortality' in Havlik RJ, Feinlieb M (eds.) *Proceedings of the conference on the decline in coronary heart disease mortality.* NIH Publication 79–1610 (Md: US Department of Health Education and Welfare, Bethesda, 1979).

13 Guberan E, 'Surprising decline of cardiovascular mortality in Switzerland', *J Epidemiol Commun Health* (1979) **33:** pp. 114–20.

14 Doll R, Peto R, 'Mortality in relation to smoking: 20 years' observation on male British doctors', *Br Med J* (1976) **2:** pp. 1525–36.

15 Schaeffer EJ, 'Premature coronary artery disease', *Primary Cardiol* (1984) **10:** pp. 151–82.

16 Kato H, Tillotson J, Nichaman MZ, Rhoads GG, Hamilton HB, 'Epidemiologic studies of coronary heart disease and stroke in Japanese men living in Japan, Hawaii and California', *Am J Epidemiol* (1973) **97:** pp. 372–85.

17 The Pooling Project Research Group, 'Relationship of blood pressure, serum, cholesterol, smoking habit, relative weight and ECG abnormalities to incidence of major coronary events. Final report of the Pooling Project', *J Chron Dis* (1978) **31:** pp. 201–306.

18 Kannel WB, 'Cigarettes, coronary occlusions, and myocardial infarction', *JAMA* (1981) **246:** pp. 871–2.

19 Townsend JL, Meade TW, 'Ischaemic heart disease risks for smokers and non-smokers', *J Epidemiol Commun Health* (1979) **33:** pp. 243–7.

20 Barboriak JJ, Anderson AJ, Hoffman RG, 'Smoking, alcohol and coronary artery occlusion', *Atherosclerosis* (1982) **43:** pp. 277–82.

21 Hartz AJ, Barboriak JJ, Anderson AJ, 'Smoking, coronary artery occlusion and non-fatal myocardial infarction', *JAMA* (1981) **246:** pp. 851–3.

22 Anonymous, 'How does smoking harm the heart [Editorial]', *Br Med J* (1980) **281:** pp. 573–4.

23 Ball K, 'Cigarettes, heart attacks and the doctor's responsibility', *Cardiol Practice* (1983) **1** (8): pp. 6–13.

24 Slone D, Shapiro S, Rosenberg L et al., 'Relation of cigarette smoking to myocardial infarction in young women', *N Engl J Med* (1978) **298:** pp. 1273–6.

25 Keys A, 'Coronary heart disease in seven countries', *Circulation* (1970) **42** (suppl 1): pp. 1–211.

26 Lewis B, 'Dietary prevention of ischaemic heart disease—a policy for the '80s', *Br Med J* (1980) **281:** pp. 177–80.

27 Gordon T, Kannel WB, Castelli WP, 'Lipoproteins, cardiovascular disease and deaths: the Framingham study', *Arch Intern Med* (1981) **141:** pp. 1128–31.

28 Berge KG, Canner PL, Hainline A, 'High-density lipoprotein cholesterol and prognosis after myocardial infarction', *Circulation* (1982) **66:** pp. 1176–9.

29 Tyroler JA, 'Epidemiology of plasma high-density lipoprotein cholesterol levels', *Circulation* (1980) **62** (suppl IV): pp. 1–136.

30 Kannel WB, Dawber TR, 'Hypertension as an ingredient of a cardiovascular risk profile', *Br J Hosp Med* (1974) **11:** pp. 508–23.

31 Castelli WP, 'Risk factors' in Sleight P, Freis E (eds.), *Hypertension* (Butterworths. London 1982), pp. 1–13.

32 Anonymous, 'Diabetes, hyperglycaemia and coronary heart disease [Editorial]', *Lancet* (1980) **i:** pp. 345–6.

33 Kannel WB, McGhee DL, 'Diabetes and cardiovascular risk factors: the Framingham Study', *Circulation* (1979) **59:** pp. 8–13.

34 Fuller JH, McCartney P, Jarrett RJ, 'Hyperglycaemia and coronary heart disease: the Whitehall study', *J Chron Dis* (1979) **39:** pp. 721–8.

35 Morris JN, Heady JA, Raffle PAB, Roberts CG, Parks JW, 'Coronary heart disease and physical activity of work', *Lancet* (1953) **ii:** pp. 1053–7, and 1111–20.

36 Paffenberger RS, Hale WE, 'Work activity and coronary heart mortality', *N Engl J Med* (1975) **292:** pp. 545–50.

37 Morris JN, Everitt MG, Pollard R, Chave SPW, Semmence AA, 'Vigorous exercise in leisure-time: protection against coronary heart disease', *Lancet* (1980) **i:** pp. 1208–10.

38 Bruce RA, 'Primary intervention against coronary atherosclerosis by exercise conditioning [Editorial]', *N Engl J Med* (1981) **305:** pp. 1525–6.

39 Gordon T, Kannel WB, 'Obesity and cardiovascular diseases: the Framingham study', *Clin Endocrinol Metab* (1976) **5:** pp. 367–75.

40 Tunstall-Pedoe H, 'Paunches and the prediction of coronary heart disease [Editorial]', *Br Med J* (1984) **288:** pp. 1629–30.

41 Mevalie JH, Goldbourt U, 'Angina pectoris among 10,000 men. II. Psychosocial and other risk factors as evidenced by a multivariate analyses of a 5 year incidence study. *Am J Med* (1976) **60:** pp. 910–21.

42 Haynes SG, Feinlieb M, Kannel WB, 'The relationship of psychosocial factors to coronary heart disease in the Framingham Study. III. Eight year incidence of coronary heart disease', *Am J Epidemiol* (1980) **III:** pp. 37–58.

43 Bass C, 'Stress personality and coronary heart disease', *Cardiol Practice* (1983) **1** (6): pp. 6–11.

44 Bass C, Wade C, 'Type A behaviour: not specifically pathogenic', *Lancet* (1982) **ii:** pp. 1147–50.

45 Marmot MG, Adelstein AN, Robinson N, Rose GA, 'Changing social class distribution of heart disease', *Br Med J* (1978) **ii:** pp. 1109–12.

46 Dimsdale JE, Hackett TP, Hutter AM, Block PC, Catanzano DM, White PJ, 'Type A behaviour and coronary angiographic findings', *J Psychosom Res* (1979) **23:** pp. 273–6.

47 Kannel WB, 'Coffee, cocktails and coronary candidates', *N Engl J Med* (1977) **297:** pp. 443–4.

48 St Leger AS, Cochrance AL, Moore F, 'Factors associated with cardiac mortality in developed countries with particular reference to the consumption of wine', *Lancet* (1979) **i:** pp. 1017–20.

49 Jick H, Meittinen OS, Neff RK, Shapiro S, Heinonen OP, Slone D, 'Coffee and myocardial infarction', *N Engl J Med* (1973) **289:** 63–7.

50 LaCroix AZ, Mead LA et al., 'Coffee consumption and the incidence of coronary heart disease', *N Engl J Med* (1986) **315:** 977–82.

51 Persky VW, Dyer AR, Idris-Sopen E et al., 'Uric acid: a risk factor for coronary heart disease?' *Circulation* (1979) **59:** pp. 969–77.

52 Mann JI, Inman WHW, 'Oral contraceptives and death from myocardial infarction', *Br Med J* (1975) **ii:** pp. 245–8.

53 Stradel BV, 'Oral contraceptives and cardiovascular disease', *N Engl J Med* (1981) **305:** pp. 672–7.

54 Khan, Kay-Tee Kaw, Peart WS, 'Blood pressure and contraceptive use', *Br Med J* (1982) **285:** pp. 403–7.

55 Gordon T, Kannel WB, Hjortland MC, McNamara PM, 'Menopause and coronary heart disease: the Framingham study', *Ann Intern Med* (1978) **89:** pp. 157–61.

57 Pocock SJ, Shaper AG, Cook DG et al., 'British Regional Heart Study: geographic variations in cardiovascular mortality and the role of water quality', *Br Med J* (1980) **1:** pp. 1243–9.

58 Larrson B, Svarddad K, Weilin L, Wilhelmsen R, Bjorntorp P, Tibblin G, 'Abdominal adipose tissue distribution, obesity and risk of cardiovascular disease and death: 13 year follow up of participants in the study of men born in 1913', *Br Med J* (1984) **288:** pp. 1401–4.

Chapter 3

1   Shaper AG, Pocock SJ, Walker M, Phillips AN et al., 'Risk factors for ischaemic heart disease: the prospective phase of the British Regional Heart Study', *J Epidemiol Commun Health* (1985) **39**: pp. 197–209.

2   Doll R, Peto R, 'Mortality in relation to smoking: 20 years' observations on male British doctors', *Br Med J* (1976) **2**: pp. 1525–36.

3   Oliver MF, 'Strategies for preventing and screening for coronary heart disease', *Br Heart J* (1985) **54**: pp. 1–2.

4   Consensus Conference, 'Lowering blood cholesterol to prevent heart disease', *JAMA* (1985) **253**: pp. 2080–6.

5   Lipid Research Clinic Coronary Primary Prevention Trial, 'I Reduction in incidence of coronary heart disease. II The relationship of reduction in incidence of coronary heart disease to cholesterol lowering', *JAMA* (1984) **251**: pp. 351–74.

6   Report from the Committee of Principal Investigators, 'A cooperative trial in the primary prevention of ischaemic heart disease using clofibrate', *Br Heart J* (1978) **10**: pp. 1069–118.

7   Turpeinen O, Karvonen MJ, Pekkarinen M et al., 'Dietary prevention of coronary heart disease: the Finnish Mental Hospital study', *Int J Epidemiol* (1979) **8**: pp. 99–118.

8   Dayton S, Pearce ML, Hashimoto S, Dixon WJ, Tomiyasu U, 'A controlled clinical trial of a diet high in unsaturated fat in preventing complications of atherosclerosis', *Circulation* (1969) **40** (suppl 2): pp. 1–63.

9   Glomsett JA, 'Fish, fatty acids and human health', *N Engl J Med* (1985) **312**: pp. 1253–4.

10   Medical Research Council Working Party, 'MRC trial of treatment of mild hypertension: principal results', *Br Med J* (1985) **291**: p. 97.

11   Amery A, Birkenhäger W, Brixko R et al., 'Mortality and morbidity from the European working party on high blood pressure in the elderly trial (EWPHE)', *Lancet* (1985) **i**: pp. 1349–54.

Chapter 4

1   Heberden W, 'Some account of a disorder of the breast. Read at the College of Physicians July 21 1768', *Medical Transactions College of Physicians* (1772) **2**: pp. 59–67.

2   Wall J, 'A letter to Dr Heberden. Read at the College of Physicians Nov 17 1772', *Medical Transactions College of Physicians* (1785) **3**: pp. 12–24.

3   Fothergill J, 'Further account of the angina pectoris', *Medical Observations and Inquiries* (1776) **5**: pp. 252–8.

4   Baron J, *The life of Edward Jenner* (Henry Colburn. London 1838), pp. 38–40.

5   Black S, *Clinical and pathological reports* (printed by Alexander Wilkinson. Newry and London 1819).

6   Parry CH, *An inquiry into the symptoms and causes of the syncope anginosa, commonly called angina pectoris* (printed by R Crutwell. Bath and London 1799).

Chapter 5

1   Bruschke AVG, Proudfit WL, Sones FM Jr, 'Progress study of 590 consecutive non surgical cases of coronary disease followed 5 to 9 years', *Circulation* (1973) **47**: pp. 1147–53.

2   Murphy ML, Hultgren HN, Detre K et al., 'Treatment of chronic stable angina: a preliminary report of survival data of the randomised Veterans Administration Co-operative Study', *N Engl J Med* (1977) **297**: pp. 621–7.

3   European Coronary Surgery Study Group, 'Longterm results of prospective randomised study of coronary artery bypass surgery in stable angina pectoris', *Lancet* (1982) **ii**: pp. 1173–80.

4   CASS principal investigators and their associates, 'Coronary Artery Surgery Study (CASS): a randomised trial of coronary artery bypass surgery. Survival data', *Circulation* (1983) **68**: pp. 939–50.

5 CASS principal investigators and their associates, 'A randomised trial of coronary artery bypass surgery. Survival of patients with a low ejection fraction', *N Engl J Med* (1985) **312**: pp. 1665–71.

6 Froelicher VF, Thomas MM, Pillow C, Lancaster MC, 'Epidemiologic study of asymptomatic men screened by maximal treadmill testing for latent coronary artery disease', *Am J Cardiol* (1974) **34**: pp. 770–6.

7 Rochmis P, Blackburn H, 'Exercise tests: a survey of procedures, safety and litigation experience in approximately 170,000 tests', *JAMA* (1971) **217**: p. 1061.

8 Ellestad MH, Cooke MMJ, Greenberg PS, 'Stress testing: clinical application and predictive capacity', *Prog Cardiovasc Dis* (1979) **21**: pp. 431–60.

9 Akhras F, Upward J, Jackson G, 'Increased diastolic blood pressure response to exercise testing when coronary artery disease is suspected: an indication of severity', *Br Heart J* (1985) **53**: pp. 598–602.

10 Borer JS, Kent KM, Bacharach SL, 'Sensitivity, specificity and predictive accuracy of radionuclide cineangiography during exercise in patients with coronary artery disease', *Circulation* (1979) **60**: pp. 752–80.

11 Ritchie JL, Trobaugh GB, Hamilton GW et al., 'Myocardial imaging with thallium-201 at rest and during exercise. Comparison with coronary arteriography and resting and stress electrocardiography', *Circulation* (1977) **56**: pp. 66–71.

12 Davis K, Kennedy JW, Kemp HG Jr, 'Complications of coronary arteriography from the collaborative study of coronary artery surgery (CASS)', *Circulation* (1979) **59**: pp. 1105–12.

Chapter 6

1 Schmeider R, Freidrich G, Neus H, Rudel H, Von Eiff AW, 'The influence of beta blockers on cardiovascular reactivity and type A behaviour pattern in hypertensives', *Psychosom Med* (1983) **45**: pp. 417–23.

2 Jackson G, 'Cardiovascular response to sexual arousal and orgasm', *Br J Sexual Med* (1986) **13**: pp. 8–9.

3 Thadani U, Mangori D, Parker JO, Fung HL, 'Tolerance to the effects of oral isosorbide dinitrate: rate of development and cross tolerance to glyceryl trinitrate', *Circulation* (1980) **61**: pp. 526–35.

4 Akhras F, Jefferies S, Jackson G, 'Isosorbide-5-Mononitrate-effective monotherapy in chronic stable angina', *Z Kardiol* (1985) **74** (suppl 4): pp. 16–20.

5 Anonymous, 'Transdermal nitrates: effective or not [Editorial]', *Lancet* (1985) **ii**: pp. 594–5.

6 Jackson G, Harry JD, Robinson C, Kitson D, Jewitt DE, 'Comparison of atenolol with propranolol in the treatment of angina pectoris with special reference to once daily administration of atenolol', *Br Heart J* (1978) **60**: pp. 998–1004.

7 Jackson G, Schwartz J, Kates RE, Winchester M, Harrison DC, 'Atenolol: once daily cardioselective beta blockade for angina pectons, *Circulation* (1980) **61**: pp. 555–60.

8 Jackson G, Atkinson L, Oram S, 'Reassessment of failed beta blocker treatment in angina pectoris by peak exercise heart rate measurements, *Br Med J* (1975) **3**: pp. 616–9.

9 Livesley B, Catley PF, Campbell RC, Oram S, 'Double blind evaluation of verapamil, propranolol and isosorbide dinitrate against placebo in the treatment of angina pectoris', *Br Med J* (1973) **2**: pp. 374–8.

10 Deanfield J, Wright C, Fox K, 'Treatment of angina pectoris with nifedipine: importance of dose titration', *Br Med J* (1983) **286**: pp. 1467–70.

11 Deanfield J, Wright C, Krikler S, Ribiero P, Fox K, 'Cigarette smoking and the treatment of angina with propranolol, atenolol and nifedipine', *N Engl J Med* (1984) **310**: pp. 951–4.

12 Lynch P, Dargie H, Krikler S, Krikler D, 'Objective assessment of antianginal treatment: a double blind comparison of propranolol, nifedipine and their combination', *Br Med J* (1980) **281**: pp. 184–7.

13 Kenny J, Daly K, Bergman G, Kerkez S, Jewitt DE, 'Beneficial effects of diltiazem

combined with beta blockade in angina pectoris', *Eur Heart J* (1985) **6:** pp. 418–23.

14 Chaffman M, Brogden RN, 'Diltiazem: a review of its pharmacological properties and therapeutic efficacy', *Drugs* (1985) **29:** pp. 387–454.

15 Anonymous, 'The expanding scope of coronary angioplasty [Editorial]', *Lancet* (1985) **i:** pp. 1307–8.

16 Hartzler GO, 'Complex coronary angioplasty: an alternative therapy', *Int J Cardiol* (1985) **9:** pp. 133–7.

17 CASS group, 'Comparison of coronary artery bypass surgery and medical therapy in patients 65 years of age or older', *N Engl J Med* (1985) **9:** pp. 133–7.

18 Chesebro JH, Fuster V, Elveback LR et al., 'Effect of dipyridamole and aspirin on late vein graft patency after coronary bypass operation', *N Engl J Med* (1984) **310:** pp. 209–14.

19 Anonymous, 'The internal mammary artery: the ideal coronary bypass graft. [Editorial]', *N Engl J Med* (1986) **314:** pp. 50–1.

20 Shaw PJ, Bates D, Cartlidge NEF et al., 'Early neurological complications of coronary bypass surgery', *Br Med J* (1985) **291:** pp. 1384–7.

21 Bass C, 'Psychosocial problems coronary artery bypass surgery', *Br J Hosp Med* (1986) **35:** pp. 111–6.

Chapter 7

1 Conti CR, Brawley RK, Griffith LSC et al., 'Unstable angina pectoris: morbidity and mortality in fifty-seven consecutive patients evaluated angiographically', *Am J Cardiol* (1973) **32:** pp. 745–50.

2 Moise A, Theroux P, Taeymans Y et al., 'Unstable angina and progression or coronary atherosclerosis', *N Engl J Med* (1983) **309:** pp. 685–9.

3 Maseri A, L'abbate A, Baroldi G et al., 'Coronary vasospasm as a possible cause of myocardial infarction: A conclusion derived from the study of 'preinfarction' angina', *N Engl J Med* (1978) **299:** pp. 1271–7.

4 Fuster V, Chesebro JH, 'Mechanisms of unstable angina', *N Engl J Med* (1986) **315:** 1023–5.

5 Duncan B, Futton M, Morrison SL et al., 'Prognosis of new and worsening angina', *Br Med J* (1976) **i:** pp. 981–4.

6 Mulcahy R, Daly L, Graham J, 'Unstable angina: natural history and determinants of prognosis', *Am J Cardiol* (1981) **48:** pp. 525–8.

7 Gazes PC, Mobley EM Jr, Faris HM et al., 'Preinfarctional (unstable) angina—a prospective study', *Circulation* (1973) **48:** p. 331.

8 Russell RO Jr, Rackley CE, Kouchoukos NT, 'Unstable angina pectoris: do we know the best management?', *Am J Cardiol* (1981) **48:** pp. 590–1.

9 The Holland Interuniversity Nifedipine/ Metoprolol Trial (HINT) research group, 'Early treatment of unstable angina in the coronary care unit: a randomized, double blind, placebo controlled comparison of recurrent ischaemia in patients treated with nifedipine or metoprolol or both', *Br Heart J* (1986) **56:** pp. 400–13.

10 Gerstenblith G, Ouyang P, Achuff SC et al., 'Nifedipine in unstable angina: a double blind randomised trial', *N Engl J Med* (1982) **306:** pp. 885–9.

11 Cairns JA, Gent M, Singer J et al., 'Aspirin, sulfinpyrazone, or both in unstable angina', *N Engl J Med* (1985) **313:** pp. 1369–75.

12 Lewis HD Jr, Davis JW, Archibald DG et al., 'Protective effects of aspirin against acute myocardial infarction and death in men with unstable angina: results of Veterans Administration Co-operative Study', *N Engl J Med* (1983) **309:** pp. 396–403.

13 De Feyter PJ, Serruys PW, Van den Brand M et al., 'Emergency coronary angioplasty in refractory unstable angina', *N Engl J Med* (1985) **313:** pp. 342–6.

14 Rahimtoola SH, Nunley D, Grunkemeier G et al., 'Ten-year survival after coronary bypass surgery for unstable angina', *N Engl J Med* (1983) **308:** pp. 676–81.

Chapter 8

1 Osler W, 'The Lumleian lectures on angina pectoris', *Lancet* (1910) **i**: pp. 697–702.

2 Prinzmetal M, Kennamer R, Merliss R et al., 'Angina pectoris. I. A variant form of angina pectoris', *Am J Med* (1959) **27**: pp. 375–88.

3 Bertrand ME, Lablanche JM, Tilmant PY, 'Frequency of provocated coronary artery spasm in 274 patients with chest pain [Abstract]', *Am J Cardiol* (1980) **45**: p. 390.

4 Selzer A, Langston M, Ruggeroli et al., 'Clinical syndrome of variant angina with normal coronary arteriogram', *N Engl J Med* (1976) **295**: pp. 1343–7.

5 Conti CR, Curry RC, 'Therapy of unstable angina pectoris' in Cohn PF (ed.), *Diagnosis and therapy of coronary artery disease* (Little, Brown. Boston 1979).

6 Bertrand ME, Lablanche JM, Tilmant PY et al., 'Complete denervation of the heart (autotransplantation) for treatment of severe refractory coronary spasm', *Am J Cardiol* (1981) **47**: pp. 1375–8.

7 Heupler FA, Proudfit WL, Razavi M et al., 'Ergonovine maleate provocative test for coronary arterial spasm', *Am J Cardiol* (1978) **41**: pp. 631–40.

8 Shroeder JS, 'Provocative testing for coronary artery spasm' in Shroeder FA (ed.) *Invasive cardiology* (Davis. Philadelphia 1985, pp. 83–96).

Chapter 9

1 Griepp RB, Stinson EB, Bieber CP et al., 'Control of graft arteriosclerosis in human heart transplant recipients', *Surgery* (1977) **81**: pp. 262–9.

2 Brush JE, Brand DA, Acampora D et al., 'Use of the initial electrocardiogram to predict in-hospital complications of acute myocardial infarction', *N Engl J Med* (1985) **312**: pp. 1137–41.

3 Morewood DJW, Whitehouse GH, 'The chest radiograph in acute myocardial infarction', *Br J Clin Pract* (1986) **40**: pp. 165–8.

4 Bonte FJ, Parkey RW, Graham KD et al., 'A new method for radionuclide imaging of myocardial infarcts', *Radiology* (1974) **110**: pp. 473–4.

5 Wackers FJTh, Schoot JB, Sokole EB et al., 'Non invasive visualisation of acute myocardial infarction in man with Thallium-201', *Br Heart J* (1975) **37**: pp. 741–4.

6 Daly K, Monaghan MJ, Jackson G., *Early detection of acute myocardial ischaemia and infarction by cross-sectional echocardiography.* 4th Symposium in Echocardiography. (Martinus Nijhoff. Rotterdam 1981), pp. 93–8.

Chapter 10

1 Norris RM, 'The management of acute myocardial infraction', *Medicine* (1985) **20**: pp. 841–7.

2 Vincent R, 'Resuscitation by ambulance crews', *Br Med J* (1986) *292:* pp. 1257–9.

3 Forrester JS, Diamond GA, Swan HJC, 'Correlative classification of clinical and haemodynamic function after acute myocardial infarction', *Am J Cardiol* (1977) **39**: pp. 137–41.

4 Koster RW, Dunning AJ, 'Intramuscular lignocaine for prevention of lethal arrhythmias in the prehospital phase of acute myocardial infarction', *N Engl J Med* (1985) **313**: pp. 1105–10.

5 Lown B, 'Lignocaine to prevent ventricular fibrillation: easy does it', *N Engl J Med* (1985) **313**: pp. 1154–5.

Chapter 11

1 Caldwell G, Millar G, Quinn E et al., 'Simple mechanical methods for cardioversion:

defence of the precordial thump and cough version', *Br Med J* (1985) **201:** pp. 627–9.

2 Chamberlain D, 'Ventricular fibrillation', *Br Med J* (1986) **292:** pp. 1068–70.

3 Camm AJ, 'Asystole and electromechanical dissociation', *Br Med J* (1986) **292:** pp. 1123–4.

Chapter 12

1 Nadeau RA, de Champlain J, 'Plasma catecholamines after cardiac infarction', *Am Heart J* (1979) **98:** pp. 548–54.

2 Ramsdale D, Farragher BE, Ward C et al., 'Pain relief in acute myocardial infarction by intravenous atenolol', *Am Heart J* (1982) **103:** pp. 459–67.

3 Frishman WH, Ribner HS, 'Anticoagulation in myocardial infarction: modern approach to an old problem', *Am J Cardiol* (1979) **43:** pp. 1207–13.

4 Weinreich DJ, Burke JF, Pauletto FJ, 'Left ventricular mural thrombi complicating acute myocardial infarction', *Ann Intern Med* (1984) **100:** pp. 789–94.

5 May GS, Eberlein KA, Furberg CD et al., 'Secondary prevention after myocardial infarction: a review of long-term trials', *Prog Cardiovasc Dis* (1982) **24:** pp. 331–52.

6 Lau YK, Smith J, Morrison SL, Chamberlain DA, 'Policy for early discharge after acute myocardial infarction', *Br Med J* (1980) **279:** pp. 1489–92.

7 Timmis AD, Rothman MT, Henderson MA et al., 'Haemodynamic effects of intravenous morphine in patients with acute myocardial infarction complicated by severe left ventricular failure', *Br Med J* (1980) **279:** pp. 989–92.

8 Muller JE, Turi ZG, Stone PH et al., 'Digoxin therapy and mortality after myocardial infarction', *N Engl J Med* (1986) **314:** pp. 265–71.

9 Parker J, Dhumate R, Pepper J, 'Recent experience with acute ventricular septal defect: the case for immediate surgery with restricted use of balloon pumping', *Br Heart J* (1985) **53:** pp. 669 [abstract].

10 Cheng TO, 'Incidence of ventricular aneurysm in coronary artery disease: an angiographic appraisal', *Am J Med* (1971) **50:** pp. 340–55.

11 Gatewood RP, Nanda NC, 'Differentiation of left ventricular pseudoaneurysms from true aneurysm with two dimensional echocardiography', *Am J Cardiol* (1980) **46:** pp. 869–78.

12 Keen DJM, Monro JL, Ross JK et al., 'Left ventricular aneurysm', *Br Heart J* (1985) **54:** pp. 269–72.

13 Buda AJ, Stinson EB, Harrison DC, 'Surgery for life-threatening ventricular tachyarrhythmias', *Am J Cardiol* (1979) **44:** pp. 1171–7.

14 Thadani U, Chopra MP, Aber CP, Portal RW, 'Pericarditis after acute myocardial infarction', *Br Med J* (1971) **ii:** pp. 135–7.

15 Anonymous, 'Pericardial effusion after acute myocardial infarction' [Editorial], *Lancet* (1986) **i:** pp. 1015–6.

16 Dressler W, 'The post myocardial infarction syndrome', *Arch Intern Med* (1959) **103:** pp. 28–42.

17 Weinlin L, Vedin A, Wilhelmsson C, 'Characteristics, prevalence and prognosis of post-myocardial infarction syndrome', *Br Heart J* (1983) **50:** pp. 140–5.

18 Rothkopf M, Boerner J, Stone M et al., 'Detection of myocardial infarct extension by CK-B radioimmunoassay', *Circulation* (1979) **59:** pp. 268–74.

19 De Soyza N, Meacham D, Murphy ML et al., 'Evaluation of warning arrhythmias before paroxysmal ventricular tachycardia during acute myocardial infarction in man', *Circulation* (1979) **60:** pp. 814–18.

20 Lawrie DM, Higgins MR, Godman MJ et al., 'Ventricular fibrillation complicating acute myocardial infarction', *Lancet* (1968) **ii:** pp. 523–8.

21 Ribner JH, Isaacs ES, Frishman WH, 'Lidocaine prophylaxis against ventricular fibrillation in acute myocardial infarction', *Prog Cardiovasc Dis* (1979) **21:** pp. 287–313.

22 Anonymous, 'Anti dysrhythmic treatment of acute myocardial infarction [Editorial]', *Lancet* (1979) **i**: pp. 193–4.

23 Chamberlain DA, Jewitt DE, Julian DG et al., 'Oral mexiletine in high-risk patients after myocardial infarction', *Lancet* (1980) **ii**: pp. 1324–7.

24 Ryden L, Ariniego R, Arnman K et al., 'A double-blind trial of metoprolol in acute myocardial infarction. Effects on ventricular tachyarrhythmias', *N Engl J Med* (1983) **308**: pp. 614–8.

25 Rossi PR, Yusuf S, Ramsdale D et al., 'Reduction of ventricular arrhythmias by early intravenous atenolol in suspected acute myocardial infarction', *Br Med J* (1983) **286**: pp. 506–10.

26 ISIS, 'Randomized trial of intravenous atenolol among 16027 cases of suspected acute myocardial infarction', *Lancet* (1986) **ii**: pp. 57–66.

27 Hjalmarson A, Elmfeldt D, Herlitz J et al., 'Effect on mortality of metropolol in acute myocardial infarction. A double blind randomised trial. *Lancet* (1981) **ii**: pp. 823–27.

28 Jewitt DE, Kishon Y, Thomas M, 'Lignocaine in the management of arrhythmias after acute myocardial infraction', *Lancet* (1968) **i**: pp. 266–70.

29 Dancy M, Ward D, 'Diagnosis of ventricular tachycardia in a clinical algorithm', *Br Med J* (1985) **291**: pp. 1036–8.

30 Krikler DM, Curry PVL, 'Torsade de pointes, an atypical ventricular tachycardia', *Br Heart J* (1976) **38**: pp. 117–20.

31 Keren A, Tzivoni D, Gavish D et al., 'Etiology, warning signs and therapy of torsade de pointes. A study of 10 patients', *Circulation* (1981) **64**: pp. 1167–74.

32 Meltzer LE, Kitchell JB, 'The incidence of arrhythmias associated with acute myocardial infarction', *Prog Cardiovasc Dis* (1966) **9**: pp. 50–63.

33 Chatterjee K, Harris A, Leathman A, 'The risk of pacing after infarction and current recommendations', *Lancet* (1969) **ii**: pp. 1061–4.

34 Atkins JM, Leshin SJ, Blomquist CG et al., 'Ventricular conduction blocks and sudden death in acute myocardial infarction: potential indications for pacing', *N Engl J Med* (1973) **288**: pp. 281–4.

35 Rentrop KP, Smith H, Painter L, Holt J, 'Changes in left ventricular ejection fraction after intracoronary thrombolytic therapy: results of the Registry of the European Society of Cardiology', *Circulation* (1983) **1** (suppl 1): pp. 55–60.

36 Swan HJC, 'Thrombolysis in acute evolving myocardial infarction', *N Engl J Med* (1983) **308**: pp. 1354–5.

37 GISSI, 'Effectiveness of intravenous thrombolytic treatment in acute myocardial infarction', *Lancet* (1986) **i**: pp. 397–402.

38 Simoons ML, Serruys PW, Brand MV et al., 'Improved survival after early thrombolysis in acute myocardial infarction', *Lancet* (1985) **ii**: pp. 578–81.

39 Balazs NDH, Saltrups A, Boxall J et al., 'Cardiac isoenzymes identify reperfusion during acute myocardial infarction', *Aust NZ J Med* (1983) **13**: pp. 402–3.

40 TIMI Study Group, 'The thrombolysis in myocardial (TIMI) trial. *N Engl J Med* (1985) **312**: pp. 932–6.

41 Mitchell JRA, 'Back to the future: so what *will* fibrinolytic therapy offer your patients with myocardial infarction?', *Br Med J* (1986) **292**: pp. 973–8.

Chapter 13

1 World Health Organization, *'Rehabilitation after myocardial infarction'* (WHO. Copenhagen 1985). (*Author's note*: An up-to-date comprehensive review.)

2 Bass C, 'Stress, personality and coronary heart disease', *Cardiol Pract* (1983) **1**: pp. 6–11. (*Author's note*: The most simple comprehensive review of stress and the heart.)

3 Jackson G, 'Sexual intercourse and post coronary patients', *Br J Sexual Med* (1979) **6**: pp. 44–8.

4 Wenger NK, 'Rehabilitation of the patient with myocardial infarction. Responsibility of the primary care physician', *Primary Care* (1981) **8**: pp. 491–507.

5 Cobb LA, 'Exercise: a risk for sudden death in patients with coronary heart disease', *J Am Coll Cardiol* (1986) **7**: 215–9. (*Author's note*: This issue has an excellent symposium on the athletic heart.)

6 Akhras F, Upward J, Keates J, Jackson G, 'Early exercise testing and elective coronary artery bypass surgery after uncomplicated myocardial infarction', *Br Heart J* (1984) **52**: pp. 413–7.

7 Bartlett RG Jr, 'Physiologic responses during coitus', *J Appl Physiol* (1956) **15**: pp. 469–72.

8 Masters WH, Johnson VE, *Human sexual response* (Little, Brown & Co. Boston 1966).

9 Nemec ED, Mansfield L, Ward Kennedy J, 'Heart rate and blood pressure responses during sexual activity in normal males', *Am Heart J* (1976) **92**: pp. 274–7.

10 Hellerstein KH, Friedman EH, 'Sexual activity in the post coronary patient', *Arch Intern Med* (1970) **125**: 987–99.

11 Bruce RA, Fisher LD, Cooper MN, Gey GO, 'Separation of effects of cardiovascular disease and age on ventricular function with maximal exercise', *Am J Cardiol* (1975) **34**: pp. 757–63.

12 Jackson G, 'Sexual intercourse and angina pectoris', *Br Med J* (1978) **2**: p. 16.

13 Larson JL, McNaughton MW, Ward Kennedy J, Mansfield LW, 'Heart rate and blood pressure response to sexual activity and a stair-climbing test', *Heart Lung* (1980) **9**: pp. 1025–30.

14 Fowler M, Jackson G, 'Cardiac failure: pathophysiology and therapy', *Update* (1983) **26**: pp. 197–204.

Chapter 14

1 Cooperative Study, 'Death rate among 795 patients in first year after myocardial infarction', *JAMA* (1966) **197**: pp. 906–8.

2 DeFeyter, PJ, van Eenige MJ, Dighton DH, Visser FC, 'Prognostic value of exercise testing, coronary angiography and left ventriculography 6–8 weeks after myocardial infarction', *Circulation* (1982) **66**: pp. 527–36.

3 Norris RM, Caughney DE, Deeming LW, Mercer CJ, Scott JP, 'Coronary prognostic index for predicting survival after recovery from acute myocardial infarction', *Lancet* (1970) **ii**: pp. 485–8.

4 Merrilees, MA, Scott, PJ, Norris RM, 'Prognosis after myocardial infarction: results of 15 year follow up', *Br Med J* (1984) **288**: pp. 356–9.

5 Sanz G, Castaner A, Betriv A et al., 'Determinants of prognosis in survivors of myocardial infarction. A prospective clinical angiographic study', *N Engl J Med* (1982) **306**: pp. 1064–70.

6 Battler A, Slutsky R, Carliner J et al., 'Left ventricular ejection fraction and first third ejection fraction early after acute myocardial infarction: value for predicting mortality and morbidity', *Am J Cardiol* (1980) **45**: pp. 197–202.

7 Chaturvedi NV, Walsh MJ, Evans A et al., 'Selection of patients for early discharge after acute myocardial infarction', *Br Heart J* (1974) **36**: pp. 533–5.

8 Shuster EH, Bulkley BH, 'Early post infarction angina: ischaemia at a distance and ischaemia in the infarct zone. *N Engl J Med* (1981) **305**: pp. 1101–5.

9 Sami M, Kraemer H, DeBusk RF, 'The prognostic significance of serial exercise testing after myocardial infarction', *Circulation* (1979) **60**: pp. 1238–46.

10 Theroux P, Waters DD, Halphen C et al., 'Prognostic value of exercise testing soon after myocardial infarction. *N Engl J Med* (1979) **301**: pp. 341–5.

11 Starling MR, Crawford MH, Kennedy GT, O'Rourke RA, 'Exercise testing early after myocardial infarction: predictive value for subsequent unstable angina and death', *Am J Cardiol* (1980) **46**: pp. 909–14.

12 Akhras F, Upward J, Stott R, Jackson G, 'Early exercise testing and coronary angiography after uncomplicated myocardial infarction', *Br Med J* (1982) **284**: pp. 1293–4.

13 Akhras F, Upward J, Keates J, Jackson G, 'Early exercise testing and elective coronary artery bypass surgery after uncomplicated myocardial infarction: effect on morbidity and mortality', *Br Heart J* (1984) **52**: pp. 413–17.

14 Akhras F, Upward J, Jackson G, 'Reciprocal change in ST segment in acute myocardial infarction: correlation with findings on exercise electrocardiography and coronary angiography', *Br Med J* (1985) **290**: pp. 1931–4.

15 Jennings K, Reid DS, Julian DG, '"Reciprocal" depression of the ST segment in acute myocardial infarction', *Br Med J* (1983) **287**: pp. 634–7.

16 Geltman EM, Ehsani AA, Campbell MK et al., 'The influence of location and extent of myocardial infarction on long-term ventricular dysrhythmia and mortality', *Circulation* (1979) **60**: pp. 805–14.

17 Moss AJ, Davis HT, DeCamilla J, Bayer LW, 'Ventricular ectopic beats and their relation to sudden and non sudden cardiac death after myocardial infarction', *Circulation* (1979) **60**: pp. 998–1003.

18 Epstein SE, Palmeri ST, Patterson RE, 'Evaluation of patients after acute myocardial infarction: indications for cardiac catheterisation and surgical intervention', *N Engl J Med* (1982) **307**: pp. 1487–92.

19 Mulcahy R, Hickey N, Graham IM, MacAirt J, 'Factors affecting the 5 year survival rate of men following acute coronary disease', *Am Heart J* (1977) **93**: pp. 556–9.

20 Wilhelmsson C, Vedin A, Elmfeldt D et al., 'Smoking and myocardial infarction', *Lancet* (1975) **i**: pp. 415–20.

21 Salonen JT, 'Stopping smoking and long term mortality after acute myocardial infarction', *Br Heart J* (1980) **43**: pp. 463–9.

22 Aronow WS, 'Effect of passive smoking on angina pectoris', *N Engl J Med* (1978) **299**: pp. 21–4.

23 May GS, Eberlein KA, Furberg CD et al., 'Secondary prevention after myocardial infarction: a review of long term trials', *Prog Cardiovasc Dis* (1982) **24**: pp. 331–52.

24 Case RB, Heller SS, Case NB et al., 'Type A behaviour and survival after acute myocardial infarction', *N Engl J Med* (1985) **312**: pp. 737–41.

25 Norwegian Multi-Center Study Group, 'Timolol induced reduction in mortality and reinfarction in patients surviving acute myocardial infarction', *N Engl J Med* (1981) **304**: pp. 801–7.

26 National Heart, Lung and Blood Institute, 'Co-operative trial. The beta-blocker heart attack trial', *JAMA* (1981) **246**: pp. 2073–4.

27 Frishman WH, Furberg CD, Friedewald WT, 'Beta adrenergic blockade for survivors of acute myocardial infarction', *N Engl J Med* (1984) **310**: pp. 830–7.

28 Julian DG, Prescott PR, Jackson FS et al., 'Controlled trial of sotalol for one year after myocardial infarction', *Lancet* (1982) **i**: pp. 1142–7.

29 European Infarction Study Group, 'A secondary prevention study with slow release oxprenolol after myocardial infarction', *Eur Heart J* (1984) **5**: pp. 189–202.

30 Australian and Swedish Pindolol Study Group, 'The effect of pindolol on the two years mortality after complicated myocardial infarction', *Eur Heart J* (1983) **4**: pp. 367–75.

31 Anderson JL, Rodier HE, Green LS, 'Comparative effects of beta adrenergic blocking drugs in experimental ventricular fibrillation threshold', *Am J Cardiol* (1983) **51**: pp. 1196–202.

32 Corday E, Heng MK, Meerbaum S et al., 'Derangements of myocardial metabolism preceding onset of ventricular fibrillation after coronary occlusion', *Am J Cardiol* (1977) **39**: 880–9.

33 Jackson G, Atkinson L, Oram S, 'Improvement of myocardial metabolism in coronary artery disease by beta blockade', *Br Heart J* (1977) **39**: pp. 829–33.

34 Griggs TR, Wagner GS, Gettes LS, 'Beta adrenergic blocking agents after myocardial infarction: an undocumented need in patients at lowest risk', *J Am Coll Cardiol* (1983) **1**: pp. 1530–3.

35 Norwegian Multicenter Study Group, 'Six year follow up of the Norwegian Multicenter Study on Timolol after acute myocardial

infarction', *N Engl J Med* (1985) **313:**
pp. 1055–8.

36 Olsson G, Lubsen J, Van Es G, Rehnqvist N,
'Quality of life after myocardial infarction:
effect of long term metoprolol on mortality
and morbidity', *Br Med J* (1986) **292:**
pp. 1491–3.

37 Seaman AJ, Griswold HE, Reaume RB,
'Long term anticoagulant prophylaxis after
myocardial infarction. *N Engl J Med* (1969)
281: pp. 115–9.

38 Sixty-Plus Reinfarction Study Research
Group, 'A double blind trial to assess longterm oral anticoagulant therapy in elderly
patients after myocardial infarction', *Lancet*
(1980) **ii:** pp. 989–94.

39 EPSIM research group, 'A controlled trial of
aspirin and oral anticoagulants in prevention
of death after myocardial infarction', *N Engl J
Med* (1982) **307:** pp. 701–8.

40 Mitchell JRA, 'Secondary prevention of myocardial infarction—the present state of the art.
Br Med J (1980) **280:** pp. 1128–30.

41 Anturan Reinfarction Italian Study Group,
'Sulphinpyrazone in post myocardial infarction', *Lancet* (1982) **i:** pp. 237–42.

42 Persantin Aspirin Reinfarction Trial Research
Group, 'Persantin and aspirin in coronary
heart disease', *Circulation* (1980) **62:** pp. 449–
61.

43 Aspirin Myocardial Infarction Study Research Group, 'A randomised controlled trial
of persons recovered from myocardial infarction', *JAMA* (1980) **243:** pp. 661–9.

44 Danish Study Group on Verapamil in Myocardial Infarction, 'Verapamil in acute myocardial infarction', *Eur Heart J* (1984) **5:**
pp. 516–28.

45 Wilcox RG, Hampton JR, Banks DC et al.,
'Trial of early nifedipine treatment in patients
with suspected myocardial infarction (the
TRENT study). *Br Heart J* (1986) **55:**
pp. 506P [abstract].

Chapter 15

1 Hutler AM, DeSanctis RW, Flynn T, Yeat-
man LA, 'Non transmural myocardial infarction: a comparison of hospital and late clinical
course of patients with that of matched
patients with transmural anterior and transmural inferior myocardial infarction', *Am J
Cardiol* (1981) **48:** pp. 591–601.

2 Madigan NP, Rutherford BD, Frye RL, 'The
clinical course, early prognosis and coronary
anatomy of subendocardial infarction', *Am J
Med* (1976) **60:** pp. 634–41.

3 Edson JN, 'Subendocardial myocardial
infarction', *Am Heart J* (1960) **60:** pp. 232–34.

4 Buja LM, Willerson JC, 'Clinicopathologic
correlates of acute ischaemic heart disease
syndrome', *Am J Cardiol* (1981) **47:** pp. 343–
55.

5 Raunio H, Rissanen V, Romppaneu T et al.,
'Changes in the QRS and ST segment in transmural and subendocardial myocardial infarction. A clinicopathologic study', *Am Heart J*
(1979) **98:** pp. 176–83.

6 Greenhoot JH, Reichenbach DD, 'Cardiac
injury and subarachnoid haemorrhage. A clinical, pathological and physiological correlation', *J Neurosurg* (1969) **30:** pp. 521–31.

7 Cotton DWK, Gallagher PJ, Sleet RA,
'Subendocardial infarction in two young
boys', *Resuscitation* (1984) **12:** pp. 181–5.

8 Von Knorring J, 'Post-operative myocardial
infarction: a prospective study in a risk group
of surgical patients', *Surgery* (1981) **90:**
pp. 55–60.

9 Szklo M, Goldberg R, Kennedy HL, Tonas-
cia JA, 'Survival of patients with non-transmural myocardial infarction: a population-
based study', *Am J Cardiol* (1978) **42:**
pp. 649–52.

10 Davies MJ, Woolf N, Robertson WB, 'Pathology of acute myocardial infarction with particular reference to occlusive coronary
thrombi', *Br Heart J* (1976) **38:** pp. 659–64.

11 Ward Kennedy J, 'Non-Q-wave myocardial
infarction', *N Engl J Med* (1986) **315:** pp.
451–3.

12 Gibson RS and the Diltiazem Reinfarction Study Group, 'Diltiazem and reinfarction in patients with non-Q-wave myocardial infarction', *N Engl J Med* (1986) **315:** pp. 423–9.

Chapter 16

1 Quyyumi A, Wright C, Fox KM, 'Ambulatory electrocardiographic ST segment changes in healthy volunteers', *Br Heart J* (1985) **53:** pp. 460–4.

2 Deanfield JE, Ribiero P, Oakley K et al., 'Critical analysis of ST segment changes in normal subjects: implications for ambulatory monitoring of myocardial ischaemia in patients with angina', *Am Med J Cardiol* (1984) **54:** pp. 1321–5.

3 Stern S, Tzivoni D, 'Early detection of silent ischaemic heart disease by 24-hour electrocardiographic monitoring of active subjects', *Br Heart J* (1974) **36:** pp. 481–6.

4 O'Rourke RA, 'Ambulatory electrocardiographic monitoring to detect ischemic heart disease', *Ann Intern Med* (1974) **81:** pp. 695–6.

5 Quyyumi A, Mockus L, Wright C, Fox KM, 'Morphology of ambulatory ST segment changes in patients with varying severity of coronary artery disease', *Br Heart J* (1985) **53:** pp. 186–92.

6 Gottlieb SO, Weisfeldt ML, Ouyang P et al., 'Silent ischemia as a marker for early unfavourable outcomes in patients with unstable angina', *N Engl J Med* (1986) **314:** pp. 1214–9.

7 Deanfield JE, Selwyn AP, Maseri A et al., 'Myocardial ischaemia during daily life in patients with stable angina: its relation to symptoms and heart rate changes', *Lancet* (1983) **ii:** pp. 753–8.

8 Schang SJ, Pepine CJ, 'Transient asymptomatic S-T segment depression during daily activity', *Am J Cardiol* (1977) **39:** pp. 396–402.

9 Jackson G, Harry JD, Robinson C, Kitson D, Jewitt DE, 'Comparison of atenolol with propranolol in the treatment of angina pectoris with special reference to once daily administration of atenolol', *Br Heart J* (1978) **40:** pp. 998–1004.

10 Pepine CJ, *Painless ischaemia: incidence, significance and on algorithm for management.* 2nd International Symposium on Mononitrate. Berlin, December 1986 (Boehringer Mannheim, in press).

Recommended reading: 'Silent ischaemia' in Pepine CJ (ed.) *Cardiology clinics.* (WB Saunders Co. 1986).

Chapter 17

1 Burch GE, Giles TD, Colcolough H, 'Ischemic cardiomyopathy', *Am Heart J* (1970) **79:** pp. 291–5.

2 Yatteau RF, Peter RG, Behar VS et al., 'Ischemic cardiomyopathy. The myopathy of coronary artery disease: natural history and results of medical versus surgical treatment', *Am J Cardiol* (1974) **34:** pp. 520–5.

3 McKee PA, Castelli WP, McNamara PM, Kannel WB, 'The natural history of congestive heart failure: the Framingham study', *N Engl J Med* (1971) **285:** pp. 1441–6.

4 Cohn JN, Archibald DG et al., 'The Veterans Administration Co-operative Study', *N Engl J Med* (1986) **314:** pp. 1547–52.

5 Starling EH, *The Linacre lecture on the law of the heart.* (Cambridge 1915). (Longmans Green. London 1978).

6 Chidsey CA, Braunwald E, Morrow AG, Mason DT, 'Myocardial norepinephrine concentration in man: effects of reserpine and of congestive heart failure', *N Engl J Med* (1963) **269:** pp. 653–8.

7 Thomas JA, Marks BH, 'Plasma norepinephrine in congestive heart failure', *Am J Cardiol* (1978) **41:** pp. 233–43.

8 Bristow M, Ginsburg R, Minobe W et al., 'Decreased catecholamine sensitivity and beta-adrenergic-receptor density in failing human hearts', *N Engl J Med* (1982) **307:** pp. 205–11.

9 Morgan DJR, Hall RJC, 'Occult aortic stenosis as cause of intractable heart failure', *Br Med J* (1979) **i**: pp. 784–7.

10 Roelandt J, 'Colour-coded Doppler flow imaging: what are the prospects?', *Eur Heart J* (1986) **7**: pp. 184–9.

11 Greenberg BH, Schutz R, Grunkemeier G et al., 'Acute effects of alcohol in patients with coronary heart failure', *Ann Intern Med* (1982) **97**: pp. 171–5.

12 Franciosa JA, Park M, Levine TB, 'Lack of correlation between exercise capacity and indexes of resting left ventricular performance in heart failure', *Am J Cardiol* (1981) **47**: pp. 33–9.

13 Katz AM, 'A new inotropic drug: its promise and a caution', *N Engl J Med* (1978) **299**: pp. 1409–10.

14 LeJemtel TH, Sonnenblick EH, 'Should the failing heart be stimulated?' *N Engl J Med* (1984) **310**: pp. 1384–5.

15 Packer M, Meller J, Medina N et al., 'Importance of left ventricular chamber size in determining the response to hydralazine in severe chronic heart failure', *N Engl J Med* (1980) **303**: pp. 250–5.

16 Dikshit K, Vyden JK, Forrester JS et al., 'Renal and extrarenal hemodynamic effects of furosemide in congestive heart failure after acute myocardial infarction', *N Engl J Med* (1973) **288**: pp. 1087–90.

17 Narins RG, 'Therapy of hyponatraemia', *N Engl J Med* (1986) **314**: pp. 1573–4.

18 Ghose RR, Gupta SK, 'Synergistic action of metolazine with loop diuretics', *Br Med J* (1981) **282**: pp. 1432–3.

19 Breckenridge A, 'Vasodilators in heart failure', *Br Med J* (1982) **284**: pp. 765–6.

20 Campbell S, Jackson G, 'Prazosin in chronic cardiac failure: a dose titration study and investigation of diuretic sparing properties', *Br J Clin Pract* (1984) suppl 29: pp. 34–42.

21 Aronow WS, 'Clinical use of nitrates. II. Nitrates in congestive heart failure', *Mod Concepts Cardiovasc Dis* (1979) **48**: pp. 37–42.

22 Franciosa JA, Cohn JN, 'Sustained haemodynamic effects without tolerance during long-term isosorbide dinitrate treatment of chronic left ventricular failure', *Am J Cardiol* (1980) **45**: pp. 648–54.

23 Taylor WR, Forrester JS, Magnusson P et al., 'Haemodynamic effects of nitroglycerin ointment in congestive heart failure', *Am J Cardiol* (1976) **38**: pp. 469–74.

24 Packer M, 'Vasodilator and inotropic therapy for severe chronic heart failure: passion and scepticism', *J Am Coll Cardiol* (1983) **2**: pp. 841–52.

25 Lipkin D, Poole-Wilson PA, 'Treatment of chronic heart failure: a review of recent drug trials', *Br Med J* (1985) **291**: pp. 993–6.

26 Packer M, Medina N, Yushak M, 'Role of the renin–angiotensin system in the development of haemodynamic and clinical tolerance to long-term prazosin therapy in patients with severe chronic heart failure', *J Am Coll Cardiol* (1986) **7**: pp. 671–80.

27 Chatterjee K, Drew D, Parmley WW, 'Combination vasodilator therapy for severe chronic congestive heart failure', *Ann Intern Med* (1976) **85**: pp. 467–70.

28 Fitchett DH, Neto JA, Oakley CM et al., 'Hydralazine in the management of left ventricular failure', *Am J Cardiol* (1979) **44**: pp. 303–9.

29 Packer M, Meller J, Medina N et al., 'Hemodynamic characterisation of tolerance to long-term hydralazine therapy in severe chronic heart failure', *N Engl J Med* (1982) **306**: pp. 57–62.

30 Cleland JGF, Dargie HJ, Hodsman GP et al., 'Captopril in heart failure. A double-blind controlled trial', *Br Heart J* (1985) **52**: pp. 530–5.

31 Francoisa JA, Wilen MM, Jordan RA, 'Effect of enalapril, a new angiotensin-converting enzyme inhibitor in a controlled trial in heart failure', *J Am Coll Cardiol* (1985) **5**: pp. 101–7.

32 Furberg C, Yusuf S, Topic N, 'Potential for altering the natural history of congestive heart failure: need for large clinical trials [Abstract]', *Am J Cardiol* (1985) **55**: pp. 45A–47A.

33 Cleland J, Semple P, Hodsman P et al.,

'Angiotensin II levels hemodynamic and sympathoadrenal function after low-dose captopril in heart failure', *Am J Med* (1984) **77:** pp. 880–6.

34 Cleland JGF, Dargie HJ, McAlpine H et al., 'Severe hypotension after first dose of enalapril in heart failure', *Br Med J* (1985) **291:** pp. 1309–12.

35 Edwards CRW, Padfield PL, 'Angiotensin-converting enzyme inhibitors: past, present and future', *Lancet* (1985) **i:** pp. 30–34.

36 Packer M, Hung Lee W, Medina N, 'Comparative effects of two converting enzyme inhibitors on renal function in patients with severe chronic heart failure: A prospective randomised clinical trial [Abstract]', *J Am Coll Cardiol* (1986) 7 (suppl A): p. 70.

37 Elkayam V, Weber L, McKay CR, Rahimtoola SH, 'Differences in haemodynamic responses to vasodilatation due to calcium channel antagonism with nifedipine and direct-acting agonism with hydralazine in chronic refractory heart failure', *Am J Cardiol* (1984) **54:** pp. 126–31.

38 Schwartz A, Allen JC, Harigaya S, 'Possible involvement of cardiac Na$^+$, K$^+$-adenosine triphosphatase in the mechanism of action of cardiac glycosides', *J Pharmacol Exp Ther* (1969) **168:** pp. 31–41.

39 Gillis RA, Raines A, Sohn YJ et al., 'Neuroexitatory effects of digitalis and their role in the development of cardiac arrhythmias', *J Pharmacol Exp Ther* (1972) **183:** pp. 154–68.

40 Withering W, *An account of the foxglove and some of its uses, with practical remarks on dropsy and other diseases* (GGJ and J Robinson. London 1785): X and V.

41 Moysey JO, Jaggarao NSV, Grundy EN, Chamberlain DA, 'Amiodarone increases plasma digoxin concentrations', *Br Med J* (1981) **282:** p. 272.

42 Johnston GD, 'Alternatives to digitalis glycosides in heart failure', *Br Med J* (1985) **290:** pp. 803–4.

43 Chamberlain DA, 'Digitalis: where are we now?', *Br Heart J* (1985) **54:** pp. 227–33.

44 Poole-Wilson PA, 'The role of digitalis in the future', *Br J Clin Pharmacol* (1984) **18:** pp. 1515–65.

45 Dollery CT, Corr L, 'Drug treatment of heart failure', *Br Heart J* (1985) **54:** pp. 234–42.

46 Taggart AJ, Johnston GD, McDevitt DG, 'Digoxin withdrawal after cardiac failure in patients with sinus rhythm', *J Cardiovasc Pharmacol* (1983) **5:** pp. 229–34.

47 Lee DC-S, Johnson RA, Bingham JB et al., 'Heart failure in outpatients. A randomised trial of digoxin versus placebo', *N Engl J Med* (1982) **306:** pp. 699–705.

48 Chamberlain DA, White RJ, Howard MR, Smith TW, 'Plasma digoxin concentrations in patients with atrial fibrillation', *Br Med J* (1970) **3:** pp. 429–32.

49 Croxson MS, Ibbertson HK, 'Serum digoxin in patients with thyroid disease', *Br Med J* (1975) **3:** pp. 566–8.

50 Wilkins MR, 'Digoxin—an update', *Prescribers J* (1986) **26:** pp. 58–65.

51 George CF, 'Interactions with digoxin: more problems', *Br Med J* (1982) **284:** pp. 291–2.

52 Aronson JK, 'Digitalis intoxication', *Clin Sci* (1983) **64:** pp. 253–28.

53 George CF, 'Digitalis intoxication: a new approach to an old problem', *Br Med J* (1983) **286:** pp. 1533–4.

54 Shapiro W, 'Correlative studies of serum digitalis levels and the arrhythmias of digitalis intoxication', *Am J Cardiol* (1978) **41:** pp. 852–9.

55 Hagemeijer F, Van Houwe E, 'Titrated energy conversion of patients on digitalis', *Br Heart J* (1975) **37:** pp. 1303–7.

56 Smith TW, Butler VP, Haber E et al., 'Treatment of life threatening digitalis intoxication with digoxin-specific Fab antibody fragments', *N Engl J Med* (1982) **307:** pp. 1357–62.

57 Leier CV, Huss P, Lewis RF, Unverferth DV, 'Drug induced conditioning in congestive heart failure', *Circulation* (1982) **65:** pp. 1382–7.

58 Scholz H, 'Inotropic drugs and their mechanism of action', *J Am Coll Cardiol* (1984) **4:** pp. 389–97.

59 Anonymous, 'Beta-agonists and heart failure [Editorial]', *Lancet* (1983) **ii:** pp. 1063–4.

60 Colucci WS, Wright RF, Braunwald E, 'New positive inotropic agents in the treatment of congestive heart failure', Part 1 and 2: *N Engl J Med* (1986) **314:** pp. 290–9 and 349–58.

61 Alderman J, Grossman W, 'Are beta-adrenergic blocking drugs useful in the treatment of dilated cardiomyopathy?' *Circulation* (1985) **71:** pp. 854–7.

62 Taylor SH, Silke B, 'Haemodynamic effects of beta blockade in ischaemic heart failure', *Lancet* (1981) **ii:** pp. 835–7.

63 Detry JMR, Decoster PM, Brausseur LA, 'Haemodynamic effects of corwin (ICI 118587) a new cardioselective beta adrenoceptor partial agonist', *Eur Heart J* (1983) **4:** pp. 584–91.

64 Anonymous, 'Ultrafiltration and haemofiltration for refractory congestive cardiac failure [Editorial]'. *Lancet* (1986) **i:** pp. 1193.

65 Kunis R, Greenberg H, Yeoh CB et al., 'Coronary revascularisation for recurrent pulmonary oedema in elderly patients with ischaemic heart disease and preserved ventricular function', *N Engl J Med* (1985) **313:** pp. 1207–10.

66 Pennoch JL, Reitz BA, Beiber CP, Stinson EG, 'Cardiac transplantation in perspective for the future', *J Thorac Cardiovasc Surg* (1982) **83:** pp. 168–77.

67 Mai FM, McKenzie FN, Kostuk WJ, 'Psychiatric aspects of heart transplantation: pre-operative evaluation and post-operative sequelae', *Br Med J* (1986) **292:** pp. 311–3.

Chapter 18

1 Kemp HG Jr, Vokonas PS, Cohn PF, Gorlin R, 'The anginal syndrome associated with normal coronary arteriograms: report of a six year experience', *Am J Med* (1973) **54:** pp. 735–42.

2 Marchandise B, Bourassa MG, Chaitman BR, Lesperance J, 'Angiographic evaluation of the natural history of normal coronary arteries and mild coronary atherosclerosis', *Am J Cardiol* (1978) **41:** pp. 216–20.

3 Jackson G, Richardson PJ, Atkinson L, Armstrong P, Oram S, 'Angina with normal coronary arteriograms: value of coronary sinus lactate estimation in diagnosis and treatment', *Br Heart J* (1978) **60:** pp. 976–8.

4 Boudoulas H, Cobb TC, Leighton RF, Wilt SM, 'Myocardial lactate production in patients with angina-like chest pain and angiographically normal coronary arteries and left ventricle', *Am J Cardiol* (1974) **34:** pp. 501–5.

5 Proudfit WL, Bruschke AVG, Sones PM, 'Clinical course of patients with normal or slightly or moderately abnormal coronary arteriograms: 10 year follow up of 521 patients', *Circulation* (1980) **62:** pp. 712–7.

6 Ockene IS, Shay MJ, Alpert JS, Weiner BH, Dalen JE, 'Unexplained chest pain in patients with normal coronary arteriograms. A follow up study of functional status', *N Engl J Med* (1980) **303:** pp. 1249–52.

7 Isner JM, Salem DN, Banas JS, Levine HJ, 'Long-term clinical course of patients with normal coronary arteriography: follow up study of 121 patients with normal or near-normal coronary arteriograms. *Am Heart J* (1981) **102:** pp. 645–53.

8 Bass C, Wade C, Hand D, Jackson G, 'Angina with normal and near-normal coronary arteriograms: clinical and psychosocial state 12 months after angiography', *Br Med J* (1983) **287:** pp. 1505–8.

9 Lavey EB, Winkle RA, 'Continuing disability of patients with chest pain and normal coronary arteriograms', *J Chronic Dis* (1979) **32:** pp. 191–6.

10 Faxon DP, McCabe CH, Kreigel DE, Ryan TJ, 'Therapeutic and economic value of a normal coronary arteriogram', *Am J Med* (1982) **73:** pp. 500–5.

11 Richardson PJ, Livesley B, Oram S, Olsen EG, Armstrong P, 'Angina pectoris with normal coronary arteries: transvenous myocardial biopsy in diagnosis', *Lancet* (1974) **ii:** pp. 677–80.

12 Rider AK, Billingham ME, Harrison DC, 'Small vessel coronary disease: biopsy evidence of intramyocardial arteriopathy', *Circulation* (1974) **50** (suppl III): p. 109.

13 Eliot RS, Bratt G, 'The paradox of myocardial ischaemia in young women with normal coronary arteriograms', *Am J Cardiol* (1969) **23:** pp. 633–8.

14 Richardson PJ, Atkinson L, Jackson G, In: Carlson LA et al. (eds). *Myocardial ischaemia and its relationship to coronary arterial disease: investigation of angina pectoris with normal coronary arteries.* International conference on atherosclerosis. (Raven Press. New York 1978), pp. 71–4.

15 Beton DC, Brear SG, Edwards JD, Leonard JC, 'Mitral Valve Prolapse: an assessment of clinical features, associated conditions and prognosis', *Q J Med* (1983) **206:** pp. 150–64.

16 Bennett JR, 'Chest pain: heart or gullet?' *Br Med J* (1983) **286:** pp. 1231–2.

17 Bass C, Wade C, Gardner WN et al., 'Unexplained breathlessness and psychiatric morbidity in patients with normal and abnormal coronary arteriograms', *Lancet* (1983) **i:** pp. 605–9.

18 Alban Davies H, Jones DB, Rhodes J, 'Esophageal angina as the cause of chest pain'. *JAMA* (1982) **248:** pp. 2274–8.

19 de Caestecker JS, Blackwell JN, Brown J, Heading RC, 'The oesophagus as a cause of recurrent chest pain: which patients should be investigated and which tests should be used', *Lancet* (1985) **ii:** pp. 1143–6.

20 Channer KS, 'Oesophageal abnormalities in patients with chest pain', *Lancet* (1986) **i:** pp. 42–3.

21 Anonymous, 'Angina and oesophageal disease [Editorial]', *Lancet* (1986) **i:** pp. 191–2.

22 Alban Davies H, Page Z, Rush EM et al., 'Oesophageal stimulation lowers exertional angina threshold', *Lancet* (1985) **i:** pp. 1011–4.

23 Bass C, Wade C, 'Chest pain with normal coronary arteries: a comparative study of psychiatric and social morbidity', *Psychol Med* (1984) **14:** pp. 51–61.

24 Bass C, Gardner WN, 'Respiratory and psychiatric abnormalities in chronic symptomatic hyperventilation', *Br Med J* (1985) **i:** pp. 1387–90.

25 Freeman LJ, Nixon PGF, 'Are coronary artery spasm and progressive damage to the heart associated with the hyperventilation syndrome?' *Br Med J* (1985) **291:** pp. 851–2.

26 Marcus ML, White CW, 'Coronary flow reserve in patients with normal coronary angiograms', *J Am Coll Cardiol* (1985) **6:** pp. 1254–6.

27 Wielgoss AT, Fletcher RH, McCants CB et al., 'Unimproved chest pain in patients with minimal or no coronary disease: a behavioural problem', *Am Heart J* (1984) **108:** pp. 67–72.

Chapter 19

1 Kleiger RE, Martin TF, Miller JP et al., Ventricular tachycardia and ventricular extrasystoles during the late recovery phase of myocardial infarction', *Am J Cardiol* (1974) **33:** p. 149 [abstract].

2 Moss AJ, DeCamilla JJ, Davies H et al., 'Use and limitations of ventricular premature beats as prognostic indicators of posthospital course of myocardial infarction', *Am J Cardiol* (1976) **37:** p. 158 [abstract].

3 De Busk RF et al., 'Serial ambulatory electrocardiography and treadmill exercise testing after uncomplicated myocardial infarction', *Am J Cardiol* (1980) **45:** pp. 547–54.

4 Lown B, Wolf M, 'Approaches to sudden death from coronary heart disease', *Circulation* (1971) **44:** pp. 130–42.

5 Moss AJ, Davis HT, DeCamilla JJ, 'Ventricular ectopic beats and their relation to sudden and non sudden cardiac death after myocardial infarction', *Circulation* (1979) **60:** pp. 998–1003.

6 Graboys TB, Lown B, Podrid J et al., 'Long-term survival of patients with malignant ventricular arrhythmias treated with antiarrhythmic drugs', *Am J Cardiol* (1982) **50:** pp. 437–43.

7 Velebit V, Podrid P, Lown B et al., 'Aggravation and provocation of ventricular arrhythmias by antiarrhythmic drugs', *Circulation* (1982) **65:** pp. 886–90.

8 Hillis WS, Whiting B, 'Antiarrhythmic drugs', *Br Med J* (1983) **286:** pp. 1332–6.

9 Vaughan-Williams EM, 'Classification of antiarrhythmic drugs' in Sandboë E, Flensted-Jensen E, Olesen KH (eds.), *Symposium on cardiac arrhythmias* (AB Astra, 1970), Södertälje, Sweden, pp. 449–72.

10 Mason W, Winkle RA, 'Accuracy of the ventricular tachycardia-induction study for predicting long-term efficacy and inefficiency of antiarrhythmic drugs', *N Engl J Med* (1980) **303:** pp. 1073–7.

11 Morady F, Scheinman MM, Hess DS et al., 'Electrophysiologic testing in the management of survivors of out-of-hospital cardiac arrest', *Am J Cardiol* (1983) **51:** pp. 85–9.

12 Ricks WB, Winkle RA, Shumway NE et al., 'Surgical management of life-threatening ventricular arrhythmias in patients with coronary artery disease', *Circulation* (1977) **56:** pp. 38–42.

13 Mason JW, Stinson E, Winkle RA et al., 'Relative efficacy of blind left ventricular aneurysm resection for the treatment of recurrent ventricular tachycardia', *Am J Cardiol* (1982) **49:** pp. 241-8.

14 Horowitz LN, Harken AH, Kastor JA, 'Ventricular resection guided by epicardial and endocardial mapping for treatment of recurrent ventricular tachycardia', *N Engl J Med* (1980) **302:** pp. 589–93.

15 Salerno JA, Klersy C et al., 'Ventricular tachycardia in post-myocardial infarction patients. Preoperative and intraoperative mapping', *Eur Heart J* (1986) 7 (suppl A): pp. 157–63.

16 Vigano M, Martinelli L et al., 'Ventricular tachycardia in post-myocardial infarction patients. Results of surgical therapy', *Eur Heart J* (1986) 7 (suppl A): pp. 165–8.

17 Mirowski M, Reid PR, Winkle RA et al., 'Mortality in patients with implanted automatic defibrillators', *Ann Intern Med* (1983) **98:** pp. 585–8.

Chapter 20

1 Topkins MJ, Artusia JF, 'Myocardial infarction and surgery. A five year study', *Anesth Analg* (1964) **43:** pp. 716–20.

2 Arkins R, Smessaert AA, Hicks RG, 'Mortality and morbidity in surgical patients with coronary artery disease', *JAMA* (1964) **190:** pp. 485–8.

3 Mauney FM Jr, Ebert PA, Sabiston DC, 'Postoperative myocardial infarction: a study of predisposing factors, diagnosis and mortality in a high risk group of surgical patients', *Ann Surg* (1970) **172:** pp. 497–503.

4 Tarhan S, Moffitt EA, Taylor WF, Givliani ER, 'Myocardial infarction after general anaesthesia', *JAMA* (1972) **220:** pp. 1451–4.

5 Steen PA, Tinker JH, Tarhan S, 'Myocardial infarction after anaesthesia and surgery', *JAMA* (1978) **239:** pp. 2566–70.

6 Goldman L, 'Cardiac risks and complications of non cardiac surgery', *Ann Intern Med* (1983) **98:** pp. 504–13.

7 Cutler BS, Wheeler HB, Paraskos JA et al., 'Applicability and interpretation of electrocardiographic stress testing in patients with peripheral vascular disease', *Am J Surg* (1981) **141:** pp. 501–6.

8 Goldman L, Caldera DL, Nussbaum SR et al., 'Multifactoral index of cardiac risk in noncardiac surgical procedures', *N Engl J Med* (1977) **297:** pp. 845–50.

Sources

The Pooling Project Research Group, *J Chron Dis* 1978) **31** for Figure 2.10; The European Coronary Surgery Study Group, *Lancet* (1982) **ii** for Figure 5.5; Vincent R, *Br Med J* (1986) **292** for Figure 10.1; Merrilees MA et al., *Br Med J* (1984) **288** for Figures 14.1–14.5; Cohn JN et al., *N Engl J Med* (1986) **314** for Figure 17.1; Pennoc et al., *J Thorac Cardiovasc Surg* (1982) **83** for Figure 17.18; Graboys et al., *Am J Cardiol* (1982) **50** for Figure 19.2.

Index

Page numbers in *italic* refer to the illustrations and tables.